TRAIL OF BONES

TRAIL

OF BONES

MORE CASES FROM THE FILES OF
A FORENSIC ANTHROPOLOGIST

Mary H. Manhein

LOUISIANA STATE UNIVERSITY PRESS)I(BATON ROUGE

First printing

DESIGNER: AMANDA MCDONALD SCALLAN
TYPEFACE: ADOBE GARAMOND
PRINTER AND BINDER: THOMSON-SHORE, INC.

Library of Congress Cataloging-in-Publication Data

Manhein, Mary H. (Mary Huffman)
Trail of bones : more cases from the files of a forensic anthropologist / Mary H. Manhein.
  p. cm.
ISBN 0-8071-3104-0 (cloth : alk. paper)
1. Forensic anthropology—Louisiana—Case studies. 2. Forensic osteology—Louisiana—Case studies. I. Title.
GN69.8.M36 2005
614'.17—dc22
                                                                                    2005003409

To my grandson, Will
My greatest inspiration

THE WHEELS OF THE GODS GRIND SLOWLY,
YET THEY GRIND EXCEEDINGLY FINE.

Contents

Illustrations

Preface

Forensic anthropology is an applied specialty within the discipline of anthropology. In this medico-legal area of forensic science, physical anthropologists trained in human skeletal anatomy examine and analyze human remains in an effort to identify the dead. This specialty requires a devotion to science, the ability to remain objective, a compassionate countenance, and the tenacity of a junkyard dog focused on its target.

As a forensic anthropologist, one of the questions I am asked most often is, "What are you doing in a field like this?" I think this question comes from the recognition that I have a passion for life and for humor. In fact, humor often saves me when things around me are not very pleasant. At a young age, I wanted to be a comedian. I saw how my antics made people laugh. However, when I tried stand-up comedy, I would start laughing at my own jokes before I delivered the punch lines and usually couldn't finish the jokes. I've never been able to keep a straight face when it comes to a funny tale, so, even early on, I knew my days as a comedian would be short indeed.

I also knew that education could be the key to any career one desires. I believe that a good dose of formal education often will lead you to your calling. It did for me. When I registered the younger of my two children for kindergarten, I matriculated as a freshman at Louisiana State University (LSU). Ultimately, I chose a career that seems to be the antithesis of my love for life and humor: investigating death. Not one funny thing about it. But one of the main reasons I picked a field that deals with death on a regular basis is simple: I can do nothing to bring back the dead, but I can help provide justice for those who can no longer speak for themselves.

While working as a forensic anthropologist for more than twenty-four years, I've also remained an advocate for the victims. I examine their bones to make sense out of who they are and to try to determine what happened to them in their last few moments before death. I strive to tell their life story from their bones.

The case studies chosen for this book are all true—real stories about real people, some cases solved, others unsolved. The names of certain victims have been changed to protect their privacy and that of their families.

Acknowledgments

To all of the law enforcement agents, coroners, crime lab investigators, and laboratory specialists who daily give your hearts and souls to your jobs, I salute you, and I thank you for allowing me into your circle of confidence. Because of you, many of the cases described in this book have been solved.

To the team of specialists with whom I work daily, Eileen Barrow, Beth Bassett, and Ginny Listi: no other forensic anthropology and imaging team in the country has so much talent concentrated in one small lab. I could not do what I do without you.

To Kerry Lyle, photographer, and Mary Lee Eggart, scientific illustrator, thank you for always being there to assist us in your most extraordinarily professional manners.

To my agent, David Madden, thank you for all of your assistance.

To Louisiana State University Press, thank you for your confidence in my work. I especially thank George Roupe, my editor, for his remarkable attention to detail and for his editing style.

Finally, to my loving family, thank you for always being there.

The End of the Road

LARRY FISHER was walking home along the railroad track that day near dusk. He was in a hurry. It was getting late and he didn't want to lose the last light of day that guided him. Looking down into the tangled brush some thirty feet below the raised track, he saw what he thought was a human leg. He was so sure of it that he climbed down the access ladder nearest him to take a closer look—it was a human leg . . . and a hip . . . and a foot. He did not touch them, nor did he want to do so. The remains were in an advanced stage of decomposition, and fly larvae, or maggots, swarmed over them in the thousands. He thought someone must have been run over by a train.

It was almost 5:00 P.M. on a Saturday evening when the sheriff's office called me that day in late December. A phone call from law enforcement on the weekend was always a serious call. We all liked our days off. A set of partial human remains had been found near a railroad track and officers needed help. Could I come? Those guys knew I would always go to any scene. We had worked on so many cases together over the years that I had lost count of them. They explained where they were. Being familiar with the area, I hopped in my Jeep and took off. Over the years, I have traveled to more than 75 percent of all of the towns and cities in Louisiana, even those in remote areas of the state that, in the last fifty years, have been reduced to whistle-stops.

Arriving just before dark, I met the case detectives near the end of a short, rural road that ended just before it reached a river. Louisiana is full of rivers and bayous, and much of my work revolves around pulling people out of one or the other. This was different. To my left was a railroad track. To my right was a single row of modest homes dotted by mailboxes at the edge of the blacktop. The long line of sheriff's department and other vehicles was strung up and down the road. Some were empty. Others were occupied by detectives and crime scene personnel awaiting my arrival.

We greeted one another with the usual hello, how are you, and my cynical, half-serious remark that they better not have called me out on a Saturday evening for a dog or deer that had been run over by a train. They laughingly assured me they had not and motioned for me to follow them. Obviously, we were not yet at the scene, though we were at the end of the road. They pointed up the rise to the railroad track. "Your vehicle awaits you, madame," one of the wisecrackers said.

I replied, "You're kidding, right?" They just laughed and started toward the motorized rail car that sat on the track. That was my first close encounter with one of the little motorized cars you see going up and down railroad tracks, usually with only one person on them, and often blocking a major intersection as the car slowly passes through. By the time we boarded the car, it was black on either side of us and behind us. The lone illumination was the car's single headlight. Though the driver assured me there were no trains due along the track from the opposite direction any time soon, I was not comforted by the thought. I had ridden behind officers on four-wheelers throughout the woods of Louisiana, sped through swamps on flatboats that operate like hydrofoils as they skim the grassy marshes, and clung to the safety bar in law enforcement vehicles on high-speed chases that occasionally interrupted our scheduled travel to a death scene. However, I was not prepared for the eerie feeling I had when I made the mistake of looking out the rail car and catching a glimpse of moonlight on water more than thirty feet below. I shuttered inwardly and held onto the handrail just a little tighter.

We slowed as we passed the railroad bridge and stopped just beyond it. "Be careful," someone called out in the night as I stepped onto the tracks from the car. I understood why. On either side of the track was very little terra firma between me and the rocks below. Periodic spring flooding from the river made it necessary to raise the tracks so high. Several flashlights beamed my way and helped to guide me as I got my bearings on the bridge.

"Mary, over here," a detective called. "We want you to look at this shoe we see on the riverbank below. Look between the crossties on the bridge." I cautiously stepped on the crossties as I moved along the bridge to its center. A flashback to my childhood reminded me that I had spent the first eight years of my life next door to a railroad switchyard in southwest Arkansas. There, my brother and I had whiled away many an hour racing up and down the tracks, touching them to feel the vibration of approaching trains. We tried to guess how long it would take before the train came around the bend. Fortunately, we had a lot more solid ground on either side of us than was available at the moment. Slowly, I got down on my hands and knees and looked through the crossties at the bank below. It was like daylight with all of the officers' flashlights trained on the spot.

"Could that be evidence?" an officer asked.

"I don't know," was my reply. I skimmed the black metal walls of the bridge with a borrowed light, noting fluorescent graffiti here and there.

"Teenagers come here all the time," a faceless voice answered my silent question. "Maybe the shoe belonged to one of them," someone else echoed.

"Should we collect it?" a crime scene tech asked.

"Sure, why not?" I said. "You never know, it might be important." The low man on the totem pole was sent down the embankment.

I continued looking at the teenagers' imaginative remarks on the bridge for a moment. The lead detective interrupted my education and said, "Over here, Mary—this is what we really wanted you to look at." He pointed to what appeared to be a wadded-up piece of fabric on the tracks just beyond the bridge. In actuality, it was a pair of boxer shorts with cartoon characters on them, completely intact, but smelling of putrefaction. Maggots swarmed inside and outside the underwear, making them move up and down on the track. My antenna went up immediately, but I didn't say anything out loud. To myself I thought, "These underwear are completely intact, no tears, no nothing." The officers had sug-

gested that the person whose leg and foot lay some thirty feet below
might have been hit by a train, knocked off the tracks, and flung into the
bushes. I knew that could not happen if this was his underwear—and
who else's would have maggots swarming in them? I had seen trains, especially freight trains, that fly like bats out of hell late in the night, but
never had I witnessed or heard of one that could knock off a man's underwear without some kind of damage. Something was really wrong here.
However, I would make that call when I saw what was below.

"It's this way, ma'am," the young officer said. His light was pointed
at a ladder attached to the side of the track. It went straight down into
the night.

"You're really kidding this time, right?"

"No ma'am," he said. "The body's down there, and the only way
down tonight is to use the ladder."

I thought, "Here I go again: up the embankment, down the railroad
track, over the river, onto the ladder, and into the dark." I felt like I was
trapped in one of Berenstain's books that had taught my children and
millions of others about prepositions and various other realities of life.
Reluctantly, I made my way over to the ladder and, not very ladylike,
managed to swing my legs over the side and onto the first two rungs. For
the umpteenth time in the last few years, I realized that I just couldn't
keep putting my body though these outrageous paces, especially at night
when a normal person would be home asleep on the sofa. Most of the
guys, and they were all males that night, were about half my age. I smiled
inwardly as I watched a few of them struggle more than I. Of course, I
could safely do so by that point. I had already made it down the ladder
and onto solid earth for the first time in almost thirty minutes. I would
think about how to get back up that ladder, onto that railroad track, and
into my own vehicle when the time came. At the moment, I had more
important things to do than worry about whether I would fall and break
my neck an hour or so down the road.

Cordoned off with the usual yellow and black crime scene tape was an
area that still buzzed with a few flies not quite ready to stop laying eggs,

or ovipositing. The sun was completely gone and I knew that any minute the flies would settle down and disappear. Dr. Lamar Meek and Jeanine Tessmer, forensic entomologists, had shown in their previous research that, in Louisiana, the flies that we use as forensic markers to help us determine time since death do not lay their eggs at night.

The smell of death was exaggerated. The maggot activity was abundant. Insects crawled all over the remains in areas that were exposed. Though it was late in the year, the heat radiating from the maggots' sheer numbers could keep them warm and make them quite active even when ambient temperatures dipped below the fifty to fifty-five degrees at which the adult flies would usually stop laying their eggs.

The scene in front of me was typical in that respect, but atypical in terms of the amount of remains. I swept the flashlight's beam back and forth across the partial body: one foot; one leg, including thigh and lower leg; the entire pelvis, including both hipbones and the sacrum. The leg was covered in part by what appeared to be undamaged nylon warmups that, like the underwear, undulated with the insect activity. The hips were coming out of the nylon warmups and were almost devoid of tissue. I quickly assessed the hip: narrow sciatic notch, acute subpubic angle— male, and young. The epiphysis on the iliac crest of the hipbone was unfused, and the pubic symphysis exhibited youthful ridges.

"What do you want to do, Mary?" the lead detective asked.

"I want to map this area quickly and triangulate the map to a pair of the closest railroad support beams. Next, I want to collect insects for analysis and then bag the remains and get them out of here. The mosquitoes are bigger than bullets and we all need to go home. Have the crime scene people finished up so that I can start?"

"Yes," several spoke in unison. We worked quickly, measuring, mapping, collecting.

"What now?" someone asked after about forty-five minutes.

"Now we go home," I replied, but I added, "Something isn't right here." I reported out loud what I had only thought earlier regarding the underwear. I told them, "I would be willing to bet that the pair of underwear on the tracks up there is associated with this. Don't ask me what happened, but no train did this. We'll figure it out tomorrow. Let's get out of here."

That was one of those times that I was glad to have ten pairs of hands. We quickly finished packaging the remains and headed for the ladder. "We'll all be back tomorrow, right?" I asked. I was quite sure that, mentally, they had already given up their Sunday plans. Once more I approached the ladder. Climbing it was not the problem. The problem arose when I got to the top. Fortunately, waiting hands lifted me like a feather, almost straight off my feet and onto the tracks. I walked over to the underwear, looked at them carefully, double gloved again, and picked them up. Something told me they were a very important part of this mystery.

The railroad service car made its way back over the graffiti-covered bridge and down the track a few hundred yards to the area closest to our cars at the dead-end road. As we slid down the embankment toward our cars, a little dog barked and barked. He was positioned near the stand of yaupon bushes close to the railroad track at the edge of the road. "He's a really good watch dog," I thought, assuming he was calling a warning to anyone who came near one of the houses across the road. He bristled at us a little, but we ignored him and went our different ways. My first stop was my laboratory, where I placed the remains on hold in the cooler. My next stop was a bath and a bed.

Early the next morning, we met again at the end of the road and opted to walk down the track to our destination. It seemed much easier that morning than the night before to climb down the ladder to the area where the partial set of human remains had been found the last evening.

We spent several hours that day looking for other remains. Approximately fifty yards away from the leg and hips, closer to the river, I spotted a cranium in a lightly wooded region. Before I touched it, I hollered for crime scene personnel to flag it, help me map it, and photograph it. Almost no tissue was left on it, and only a weak scent of decomposition floated up from it. Though youthful in appearance, several of the cranial sutures, or joints, were fused, which is not that uncommon, but it did give me pause. Usually, the sutures are unfused, or open, in a person under twenty-five, as I thought the victim was. The last thing I wanted was for there to be two bodies out there if the cranium did not go with the obviously youthful hips and leg. I turned the cranium over and looked at the teeth. They were the teeth of a young adult. Also, most of the sutures in the roof of the mouth were unfused, again a sign of a relatively young person.

The square eye orbits, nasal width, and prognathic alveolar region suggested he was black, though measurements back at the lab could help to confirm that. It was the condition of the maxillary teeth, however, that surprised me. They were cracked and broken and a one-half inch section of the maxillary bone was missing. Nothing else on the cranium was damaged. The trauma was so localized that I knew a train could not have done this. Once again, another mystery was added to the story. It seemed as though everything we found added to the puzzle rather than helping us solve it.

We bagged the cranium and continued to look for more remains. I headed toward the area where the leg and hips had been found the day before. Smelling something very strong on the wind, I thought it might be the body residue left over from last night. I approached the first death scene from behind the area where we had collected the remains. Brushing aside some tall bushes, I momentarily felt I was reliving the prior evening's events. There, on some bushes in front of me, were the other leg and foot draped over a four-foot-high stand of weeds. They were only three or four yards directly behind where the first set of partial remains had rested earlier. I yelled for help.

Once again, we mapped the location of the remains, photographed them, and bagged them. The train theory was going out the window, though that had happened for me the night before. We continued looking for the rest of the body. Our effort was concentrated on the eastern border of the river on the same side of the bridge on which the remains had been found. We had gone up and down the riverbank, all through the woods, and finally had called it quits. The entomologist, Dr. Lamar Meek, had come to the scene and noted that fly activity suggested an approximate time since death of around three weeks. I agreed. Also, by the end of our search that day, local news reporters had heard about the case, and we knew it would hit the ten o'clock news. It did.

The next day, a Monday, I was unavailable for another search until late morning. Naturally, a sheriff's detective called with big news. A suspect had come forward the evening before and had confessed to the crime. He agreed to show law enforcement agents the location of the rest of the remains. Research associates Ginny Listi and Beth Bassett headed out to the scene, and I planned to meet them there after teaching my morning class. The three of us had worked together for years, and I knew they would do an outstanding job of collecting and mapping anything else that might be found. They met the officers, and the puzzle began to fit together.

At the end of the road, near where the little dog barked and barked, was a region of thick brush. The perpetrator started there to tell the detectives his story. He said he had a disagreement with the victim at another location miles away and they ended up in a fight. In self-defense, he said, he stabbed the victim in the upper left chest one time, mortally wounding him. He gave a date of approximately nine weeks prior to the discovery of the body, not three weeks as the insect activity had suggested. He noted that he had brought the victim to the region at the end of the rural road and had dragged him into the heavy underbrush across the road from the houses and near the railroad track.

For weeks afterward, he thought about the killing. He was afraid that someone would find the body so close to the houses and decided that he had to conceal it more effectively. He went out to the dump site late at night and started moving the body. Of course, after several weeks of decomposition, the body was in an advanced stage of putrefaction. He said he picked up the major parts of the body and began walking up the embankment, down the track, and toward the railroad bridge. As he did so, he dropped a few things along the way—ribs, a shoe.

As he started down the tracks, he discarded body parts. The entire vertebral column had desiccated, or dried out, by that time and had become one long set of partially mummified remains. He threw that to the left of the track as he headed east. He crossed the railroad bridge lugging his decaying victim. That was where he lost the underwear when he stopped. He stopped for a reason. He picked up the cranium, he said, and looked at the teeth. A light went off in his head. He remembered seeing on TV that you could identify someone from his teeth. With that thought in mind, he took the cranium and pounded and pounded it on the rails, cracking and breaking several teeth and part of the maxillary bone. Sure enough, crime scene personnel looked down between the crossties and saw small chips of tooth enamel among the rocks. We never would have noticed those tiny fragments without the perpetrator's help.

Then, he said, he looked to his left and saw a telephone pole. Aiming in that direction, he hurled the cranium that way, exactly where I had found it the day before. To confuse the issue even further, he turned and threw the lower jaw more than thirty yards on the other side of the track. One of the detectives who was with him during his confession had an idea. He picked up a rock that he thought might be similar in weight to a human mandible and hurled it across the high grass. A crime scene technician climbed down the ladder and made his way through the heavy brush to the approximate spot. Within three yards of that spot, he found the mandible, a true needle in a haystack.

Next, the perpetrator said, he picked up the lower body, which was coming completely apart by this time (at the spot where the underwear had been found) and walked a few more yards down the track. He threw one leg to the left side of the track and then flung the second one in the same direction—exactly where we had found them.

The discrepancy in the insect activity evaluation we had provided the day before made sense now. Actually, there were two insect infestations, one at the original dump site and a new one at the location where the assailant subsequently redeposited the body parts.

After I heard the incredible story, I walked inside the cluster of bushes where the perpetrator had first placed the body. Evidence was everywhere. Parts of the upper body were still there: scapulae, humeri, radii, and ulnae. A shirt was matted to the soil. In the upper left chest region of the shirt was a one-inch slit, most likely made by the knife the perpetrator had used. In recovering the ribs, we found that the second left rib had a one-inch perimortem cut across its inferior border, right in line with the cut area in the shirt. Beth and Ginny had finished mapping all of the bones by that time, and one could literally see a trail of bones for more than seven hundred yards. A few weeks later, or maybe even just days later, crucial evidence might have been lost.

I had been shortsighted when I concentrated my earlier search efforts on the other side of the river's bank. Though we had looked on the west side, we paid much more attention to the east side. Natural geographical barriers can prejudice a search area. Also, the cadaver dog we had used had not picked up anything in either of the two areas. I chided myself for not paying more attention to the area with the closest access by road. Our subsequent research on body dump sites has shown that the area nearest the closest access by vehicle is generally an excellent place to look for a body and to look very closely. In this case, the body had lain in the bushes immediately adjacent to the dead end road for more than six weeks.

And then the little dog: lab analysis of the remains revealed canine tooth marks across many of the bones that were found in the bushes by the road. His barking was probably to protect his stash, not his home.

However, the most telling part of this case was the perpetrator himself. His television experience with regard to teeth being valuable tools for identification was absolutely correct. It was in his other assumption that he was somewhat confused. He told the detectives the reason he confessed to the crime was that he had heard somewhere that you could get fingerprints from bones, and he knew that they would catch him anyway. Small consideration. He noted to detectives in the beginning that he was wearing his mother's rubber kitchen gloves the entire time he was disposing of the body. His confusion led to yet another research project we conducted recently with regard to fingerprints on bones. The positive results will be published shortly.

The Lady from the Gulf

I T was early July when the lady from the Gulf was brought to my laboratory. Occasionally, the mornings were still cool with a pleasant breeze from the southwest, directing the heady scent of magnolia blossoms my way and making early summer in south Louisiana almost tolerable. Spring semester had ended several weeks earlier, and all of the graduate students had gone home or were off working on their summer research projects. For a brief period, I had no papers to grade, no marathon discussions on proposed thesis topics, no deadlines for a thesis defense, and no constant knocks on my door. July was the time when my assistants and I began our own summer research and prepared for a well-earned week or two of vacation. Inevitably, however, summer was also a time when we received several calls for assistance in forensic cases.

Anthropology graduate students wait expectantly throughout the year for opportunities to participate in field retrievals and analysis of forensic cases. Yet most of the cases seem to come during the summer or between semesters when the students are gone. That's the way it was in 1999, when we were asked to consult on a case being secured at the Jefferson Parish morgue. Jefferson is a sprawling parish of more than 450,000 people. It spans both the east and west banks of the Mississippi River and encompasses, among others, the city of Metairie and other parts of greater New Orleans. The Jefferson Parish coroner's office has a large morgue facility, which is shared by other parishes that surround Jefferson, including Plaquemines Parish, a narrow peninsula a few miles south of New Orleans.

On that late spring day in 1999, Anthony Buras, senior coroner's in-

vestigator for Plaquemines Parish, called and asked if I would meet him
at Jefferson's morgue to review the case of a man they had found on the
bank of the Mississippi River the day before. Unfortunately, the Mississippi River gives up bodies on a regular basis, especially those of young
men. Though sex and probable race of this most recent victim were determined from preserved soft tissue, the autopsy had not revealed enough
information to lead investigators to a positive identification.

The identity of the young black man from the riverbank was easy
enough once we examined him in our laboratory at LSU in Baton Rouge.
Our Forensic Anthropology and Computer Enhancement Services
(FACES) Laboratory handles cases from all across the country. In the
Plaquemines case, careful examination of the decaying body revealed a
tattoo on the young man's forearm. It had been obscured by the rigid position of his limbs and the discoloration of his skin tissue resulting from
desiccation of his remains on the river's edge. "Sam," a nickname he had
used for many years, was revealed clearly when we dabbed a small
amount of diluted household bleach on the leatherlike skin. But it was
the visit to the morgue to review Sam's case that day that ultimately
brought the mystery woman to our lab. Sam's accidental death when he
fell from the boat on which he was working, while tragic in its own right,
would be a far simpler case than the one to which we were about to be
introduced.

While waiting for permission to release the river case to us, Terri Kin-
ney, coroner's investigator and morgue manager for Jefferson Parish,
asked if I would like to see a case they had autopsied earlier that year
which remained unsolved, including the identification. It is not at all unusual in our line of work to travel to a morgue for consultation on one
case and end up with multiple cases. Of course, I agreed.

This Jane Doe was found on February 4, 1999, floating in the salt water
approximately fifteen miles south of Grand Isle, Louisiana, in the Gulf
of Mexico. Grand Isle is a sleepy little fishing village of about 1,500 people that actually is a barrier island located off the tip of Louisiana's
marshy coastline—one road in, one road out. In the nineteenth century a
popular resort on the island attracted vacationers from all across the

country. Today, the hotel is long gone, any evidence of it and many other landmarks destroyed by a hurricane in 1893. However, visitors still arrive in droves, especially fishermen anxious to rent the day boats to try their hand at deep sea fishing. Though the new Jane Doe had probably been dead for less than a month when a fisherman discovered her body, the pathologist's autopsy and subsequent profile had not resulted in identification several months following her recovery.

Her face was flat and void of expression, moisture dripping from the tip of her nose. Her medium-length, brown and graying hair was slipping from the scalp that had held it in place. Her body was stitched together with thick twine. The faint odor of the ocean that recently had given her up clung to her in the cold morgue.

I stared at her for a few minutes that day in the morgue. I wondered who she was, why she had been shot in the chest, wrapped in a fishing net taped securely in place with gray duct tape, and weighted down with a forty-pound homemade concrete anchor. Whoever placed her there had expected her to sleep forever among the fishes. But sometimes the warm Gulf waters lend justice a hand, in this case allowing the body, with its gases slowly building in the gut, to rise to the surface for all to see. Her odyssey had only begun.

I thanked Terri for allowing us to view the woman's body that day. We never touch a case until we are asked to consult by the lead agency involved. In this instance, it was a matter of a phone call to the Federal Bureau of Investigation (FBI). The woman from the Gulf was an FBI case because the FBI investigates "crimes on the high seas." Barbara O'Donnell, special agent for the FBI, seemed glad to hear from me. She was not the original investigator on the case, but she noted how frustrating it had been for her not to obtain an identification on the victim since the case had been turned over to her. Without first identifying her, the FBI really had no place to start in order to find out who had killed the woman. I explained how a second examination might add additional information to a case, especially if completed by a forensic anthropologist. Agent O'Donnell agreed to transfer the body of the mysterious woman from the Gulf to the FACES Lab for further review.

The new case, numbered 99-15, our fifteenth case in 1999, was one of a growing list of more than seven hundred on which we have worked over the years, having dealt with all law enforcement agencies within our state as well as many others from across the country. Agent O'Donnell and I became fast friends with a singular goal—identification and resolution of the case from the Gulf. Her investigation of the case would carry her all across the country for years to come and land us both on national television on several occasions.

The FBI arranged for the lady from the Gulf to be transported to our laboratory. At the FACES Lab, our preliminary examination of 99-15 included a full-body x-ray. The x-ray captured small fragments of metal in her chest region. They showed up on the anterior-posterior view of her chest as white jagged specks and were most likely associated with the bullet that killed her. The entry wound for the bullet was obscured in the postautopsy tissue, but our subsequent examination of the bony elements revealed damage to other parts of her body.

Finally, we carefully checked the body bag for any additional evidence, part of our protocol in every forensic case. Over the years, our examination of postautopsy remains and the body bags in which they were placed, in addition to our mandatory x-rays, have provided law enforcement agencies with valuable information. Since finding disarticulated fingers, complete with fingerprints, that led to an elderly man's positive identification in a five-year-old burial case in one postautopsy examination, we've learned never to be surprised by evidence hidden in the putrefactive tissue of a decaying body. The often unpleasant task of meticulous examination of such material has lent itself to continuous ribbing from some law enforcement agents and, when something of significance is found, many a sheepish exclamation of newfound respect from those who rarely would venture into such territory. In the case of 99-15, our efforts were not unwarranted.

The unidentified female's preliminary x-rays were full of surprises. Not only did they expose the small metal fragments in her chest, they also highlighted her extensive dental restoration work and revealed several characteristics about her skeleton that could provide clues to her identity.

The soft tissue confirmed that the victim was a mature female, most likely of white European ancestry; however, in order to analyze her skeleton, the decaying tissue had to be removed with scalpels, sharp scissors, heated water, and mild detergent.

Once this task was completed, our metric analysis of her skull suggested her ancestry. Additionally, her skull shape offered other clues to her race. She had a small, pinched nasal opening; a narrow interorbital breadth (the distance between her eyes); a long anterior nasal spine (the small bony projection in the center of the lower border of the nasal opening); sloping, oval eye orbits; a straight, or orthonathic, profile when the skull was viewed in a lateral position; a parabolic dental arch; and a slight overbite. She was what we call "classic white European."

Two regions on her hipbones, her auricular surfaces (where the hip bones meet the sacrum) and her pubic symphysis (where the hipbones come together in the front of the body), as well as the sternal ends of her ribs, provided us with an estimate of her age: forty-eight to sixty years. Those areas on the skeleton change in appearance as an adult human ages (what we call "bone remodeling"), and the age-related changes associated with these sites have been used to establish aging standards based on the study of cadavers where true age is known.

Next, we wanted to determine her height. To do this, we measured her long bones: her femur, tibia, fibula, humerus, radius, and ulna. Only one complete long bone is essential to estimate height accurately, but we usually prefer to use the femur, or thighbone. Typically, it provides a solid estimate of height. We plugged the length of her left femur (420 millimeters) into a regression formula whose results indicated that she was between five feet two and five feet five inches tall. Her estimated living weight of approximately 125 to 135 pounds had been set at autopsy. Generally, we agreed.

There we had it, her skeletal profile: white female, forty-eight to sixty years of age, approximately five feet three inches tall, weighing around 125 to 135 pounds.

Our profile usually includes time since death—the postmortem interval, as we call it, or PMI. Since we had not viewed the body when it first came out of the Gulf, we left that assessment to the pathologist who had performed the autopsy. The original estimate was approximately two to eight weeks. Now that we had our profile, similar to what the pathologist had originally suggested, we could concentrate on the information that might help to get her identified—those many dental restorations, bony anomalies, and her personal belongings.

Though various tooth numbering systems exist, many dentists use one known as the Universal Numbering System to identify adult teeth, which are numbered 1 through 32. Beginning in the back of the mouth on the upper right, the last molar tooth (also referred to as the wisdom tooth) is designated as tooth number 1. The upper teeth are numbered sequentially from 1 to 16, ending with the third molar (wisdom tooth) on the upper left. The numbering system then drops to the lower jaw at the back of the mouth on the left side and starts with the last tooth—the third molar, or wisdom tooth. It is assigned the number 17, and the lower teeth are then numbered sequentially around to the last tooth on the lower right, number 32. This numbering system is quite useful in establishing a putative ID. Antemortem x-rays and written records of the individual's teeth can be used to confirm an identification or eliminate a person from consideration. For example, when discussing restorations or extractions, all dentists recognize tooth 8 as the upper right central incisor.

Case 99-15 had more dental work than most. She had porcelain crowns on all four of her upper central teeth, or incisors (teeth 7, 8, 9, and 10). Also, she had a porcelain crown on tooth 30 and a gold crown on tooth 15. Additionally, she had amalgam fillings in several teeth as well as composite fillings in others. Her four wisdom teeth (numbers 1, 16, 17, and 32) were missing. She may have been one of the rare individuals born without those tooth buds, but more than likely, she had her wisdom teeth removed sometime during her adult life. She retained the rest of her teeth. Drs. Robert Barsley and Ronald Carr, odontologists with whom I have worked for more than fifteen years, examined 99-15's remains and provided us with additional information regarding her dental status and health. Since both of these odontologists are professors at the LSU School of Dentistry in New Orleans, they are well versed in current as well as past techniques, preparation, and materials used for dental restorations.

Additionally, certain aspects of dentistry, including the materials used in fillings, vary throughout the world, and odontologists are able to recognize the variations. Of the 170,000 dentists in the United States, only about one hundred routinely work with law enforcement in identification of the dead.

Drs. Barsley and Carr noted that 99-15's dental work appeared to be American in origin and was typical of a middle-class socioeconomic background that included good dental care. Added to that, the appearance of the fillings suggested that several of the teeth had been repaired twenty-five to thirty years earlier.

Another morphological identifier for this woman was the large bony tori present in her jaws. A torus (plural *tori*) is a bony protrusion, or ridge of bone. In dentistry, such a protrusion can be found in multiple locations. In the roof of the mouth, many people have a long bony ridge, or torus, running down the center of their palate. You can feel it with your tongue. In the case of 99-15, tori were present in her maxilla and in her lower jaw. Those in her lower jaw were represented by fairly large outgrowths of bone on each side of her mandible protruding into the tongue, or lingual, region of her jaw. A dentist probably would have noted these in her records.

It was not just 99-15's dental profile that could help us. Her skeleton offered even more clues. On her left leg, her tibia and fibula, the long bones below the knee, showed evidence of old fractures, and our x-rays confirmed them. The fractures were fairly extensive, but both bones had been broken long enough before death for the injuries to have healed completely. The fibula, the thin outer bone, had a healed break a few inches below the knee. The tibia had a healed break near the midshaft region. Had our woman from the Gulf fallen from a horse when she was younger? Had she been in a life-threatening automobile wreck or some other devastating accident? We had no way of knowing, but a doctor's care would have been essential for these injuries. Subsequent analysis of her right leg revealed an arthritic knee with little bony growths, or spicules, on her knee cap, her patella. This suggested that in favoring her left leg, she seems to have put enough pressure on her right leg to have damaged that knee. This evidence indicated that years may have passed since she had broken her left leg. Could she have walked with a limp from these combined stress factors on both legs? Perhaps. These old injuries and her dental history were just the beginning of a tale that started to reveal itself.

Clearly, our lady from the Gulf was dressed for winter on her ill-fated day. Her clothing was casual, an acrylic sweater and pull-on knit pants, most likely dark blue in color. The sweater was a pullover with a pocket on the left side over the breast region. The pocket had a decorative nautical appearance, with a fleur-de-lis and horizontal and slanted stripes. The blue sweater's label read "David Benjamin, Size Medium, DB Sport." Over that she wore a bulky, cable-knit sweater. She had on boots and heavy socks.

After weeks of searching for the sources of her clothing, the FBI investigators traced her blue sweater to the Lerner Shop, a popular, moderately priced clothing store that has been in business for many years. Representatives from Lerner noted they had not made that particular style of clothing since the early 1990s. Her boots were still on her feet when she was recovered and were brown, ankle high, lined, leather-suede with molded synthetic soles. "Thom McCann" was on the label and the boots were "size 5." Again, Thom McCann had not manufactured those particular boots since the early '90s.

Her thick outer sweater she had worn to keep out the winter chill of the Gulf waters had no label. Most likely homemade, the bulky, cable-knit garment had a rolled collar and no buttons. It may have been worn loosely or had a tie around the waist. Several possibilities existed for the sweater. She may have knitted it herself, it may have been a gift, or it and the rest of her clothing might have been purchased at a garage sale or second-hand clothing store. In such cases, we always have to remember that clothing items may have been recycled.

In addition to distinctive clothing, 99-15 wore two pieces of jewelry—a plaited gold or gold-plated bracelet around her wrist and an unusual necklace. The necklace offered possibilities for identifying her (FIGURE 1). It was a butterfly pendant approximately one inch in length and width. The wings of the butterfly appeared to be small diamond chips set in a gold base. The body of the butterfly was an elongated blue stone

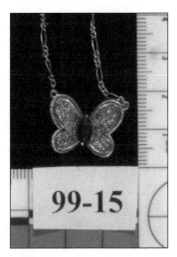

FIGURE I.
Necklace of the Lady from the Gulf

(lapis lazuli). The butterfly was attached to the gold chain by a loop at the top of each wing. Yancy Guerin, a coroner's investigator for West Baton Rouge Parish and a victims' advocate, conducted an Internet search for like jewelry. He found a similar necklace, but it was not an exact match. The source of her necklace remained unknown. One might argue that the necklace also could have been recycled. However, something about the smooth appearance of the back of the butterfly suggested that the necklace was a well-loved piece of jewelry 99-15 may have worn regularly for a long time.

Then there was the fishing net. Agent O'Donnell traced the net to a company in the northeastern United States. The company's distribution center noted that those particular nets were sold all across the country and even in some foreign countries. The fishing net provided no clues. Neither did the homemade concrete anchor. Weighing approximately forty pounds with a large metal loop at the top, it has not been traced to its source.

Finally, 99-15's location in the ocean might offer clues. Fifteen miles out in the Gulf was getting into really deep water said Dr. Gregory Stone, chairman of LSU's Department of Coastal Studies and an internationally recognized expert on the Gulf coast. He explained, "January and February can be very rough in the Gulf, Mary. Strong winds from the south contribute to what are called 'prefrontals,' and waves can be as high as fifteen feet."

My main question for Dr. Stone was about the possibility of transport. "Could she have come from some other country, say Cuba or Mexico?" I asked. Dr. Stone agreed with me that the forty pounds attached to her body and her particular location in the Gulf suggested that she was probably placed in the water somewhere in the general vicinity of where she was found. He also agreed that whoever placed her there thought he was far enough out from shore to be safe from discovery. Finally, Dr. Stone noted that the usually warm Gulf waters were fairly cool at that time of year, typically fifty to fifty-five degrees.

In my experience with bodies found in water, even cool water, if the person has drowned, initially the body sinks. After a few hours, it may rise to the surface if not trapped by some means. When it rises to the surface, sometimes the person will be face down with the back showing just above the water's surface and the limbs dangling below. At other times, the body will be face up with the limbs floating slightly below the surface. Furthermore, dangling body parts with mobile joints are attractive to marine life and often are the first to be lost: the hands, the feet, the head. In this case, the net with its tape prevented that from happening. Also, the forty-pound homemade concrete anchor attached to 99-15's small body impeded its rise to the surface, delaying it for days or even weeks. Correspondingly, the cool temperature of the water at that time of year would have slowed the decomposition process, making it more difficult to estimate time since death. Eventually, however, as the inevitable decomposition processes began to occur, the body became buoyant and floated, in spite of the weight attached to it.

With most other resources exhausted in the search for the identity of 99-15, we decided to reconstruct her face in order to have a proper image for the public to view for possible identification. Eileen Barrow, forensic artist and sculptor at the FACES Laboratory, began to work her magic in clay. First, she anchored the real skull to a metal rod that was positioned on a wooden base. Then she padded the back of the fragile eye orbits and nasal opening with cotton to protect them from harm. Next, she glued twenty-one small tissue depth markers directly onto the skull. The tissue depth markers, cut to precise lengths in millimeters, help to determine the average tissue thickness at strategic points across the face. For example, most people have somewhere between four and five millimeters of tissue thickness in the center of their forehead between their eyes.

Allowing the glue beneath the markers time to dry, Eileen then anchored the prosthetic eyes in the orbits. The shape of the person's eye orbits dictates whether the eyes will be deep set, even with the outer borders of the eye orbits, or slightly projecting. Next, Eileen measured the maximum width of the nasal opening to help determine the breadth of the lower nose. The length of the nose was established in part by measuring the small bony projection, or anterior nasal spine, at the base of the nose and incorporating that measurement into a formula designed to help in shaping the nose. Finally, she determined the fullness of the lips from the measurement taken from the top gum line to the bottom gum line in the center of the mouth. Usually, the width of the mouth stretches from canine tooth to canine tooth.

To create a realistic image of 99-15, Eileen manually added clay across the skull and filled in all features of the face. Once this was completed, she photographed the image, scanned that photograph into a computer file, and completed her final finishing work on the image in Photoshop, a computer software package used by some forensic artists and sculptors to finesse their reconstructions. The clay image of 99-15 is presented in FIG-URE 2. We always note in such cases that the idea behind a facial reconstruction is not to create an exact likeness of the victim but to construct an image that might jog someone's memory. Science and artistic license come together in this process, but care should be taken so that artistic license does not supersede the science behind the technique.

In order to generate public attention for this case, Agent O'Donnell and I appeared on television stations in New Orleans on multiple occasions. We also participated in a special on the Discovery Channel to appeal to the public to help us identify the mysterious woman found floating in the Gulf of Mexico. Additionally, 99-15 received a brief mention on national television in the spring of 2004 when I was asked to com-

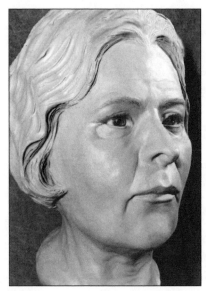

FIGURE 2.
Clay image of the Lady from the Gulf

ment on the case of a woman and child found floating in San Francisco Bay. That young woman and her child were subsequently identified.

Never in the history of our laboratory had we had such an extensive profile on a person and not been able to provide a positive identification. I believed we would get our lady from the Gulf identified, either from her fingerprints, the DNA extracted from her bones, her broken and healed lower left leg, her extensive dental work, her unusual butterfly necklace, or perhaps her facial reconstruction. Agent O'Donnell and I awaited the phone call that would lead to her identity. Whoever dumped 99-15 in the Gulf of Mexico did not expect her to rise like a phoenix. That was his or her first mistake.

In October 2004, more than five years after 99-15's body was discovered in the Gulf of Mexico, Drs. Robert Barsley and Ronnie Carr were provided dental records of a sixty-five-year-old woman who was last seen on or around January 11, 1999. She had been reported missing from Missouri. After years of searching for her identity, the phone call Agent O'Donnell and I had been hoping for finally came. An unusual name on a tag sewn into a piece of her clothing was traced to a relative's married name. My role in this case was finished. That of law enforcement had just started.

Coming Home

I N the summer of 2003, I watched the backhoe from the shade of a sweet gum tree at the edge of a small cemetery in southern Arkansas. For some strange reason, the words to "When Johnny Comes Marching Home" kept running silently through my head. The young man in the grave we were exhuming had come home some forty-eight years earlier, but he had not been marching at the time. Corporal James B. Sanders, Company D, 32nd U.S. Infantry Regiment, was just nineteen years old when he died during the Korean War. Of course, officially, it was not a war, just a conflict, but U.S. soldiers died by the thousands just the same. For the second or third time in as many weeks, I asked myself once again why was I involved in this case. My thoughts slipped backward almost a year to my initial introduction to the Sanders family.

In July 2002, I was contacted by Shelley Belgard, a victims' advocate who had been working with various families of POWs and missing soldiers from several wars. Shelley herself had a missing uncle from one of the wars. She had heard about my work on historic cemeteries and forensic burials and called to ask if I would be willing to help the Sanders family. She related their story to me.

Corporal Sanders's mother was in her nineties at the time and in poor health, Shelley said. Since "Jim" had been sent home all those long years ago, his mother had been troubled greatly about whether or not the remains in the casket were actually his. The usual rumors had also circulated, arousing suspicion in some, that sealed caskets from that era might not have any bones at all in them. Corporal Sanders's remains had been returned to U.S. custody by communist forces years after he had been reported missing in the Chosin Reservoir of Korea during a mission on December 2, 1950. Though the remains identified as Corporal Sanders's had been buried in Arkansas in 1955, his name continued to be listed on official government rolls as being unaccounted for as late as 1957. Lloyd Sanders, Corporal Sanders's older brother and the family spokesperson, wanted to provide peace of mind for his mother and ease the doubt she and the rest of the family had felt over the years. Lloyd, too, was a soldier during the Korean War, but the army had not allowed him to come home for his baby brother's funeral, another reason for distrust.

War does strange things to people. Sealed caskets sometimes lend doubt to the veracity of government papers. Additionally, the army was not interested in getting involved in the Sanders family's investigation. Though polite, army officials were steadfast, and understandably so, in their decision to stay away from any effort to exhume a body that had already been identified or to try to second-guess an identification made almost fifty years earlier. They advised the family, however, that the army could do nothing to stop them if they wished to pursue their inquiry.

It was not just the sealed casket or government lists that bothered the Sanders family. A seemingly minor detail had been nagging at them in the years since they had received the documents describing Corporal Sanders's body. The official government report noted that on December 2, 1950, Corporal Sanders (at that time Private Sanders) was part of an effort in enemy territory in the Chosin Reservoir region of Korea to secure the town of Hagaru-ri. He was reported missing that day. Years later, his skeletal remains and those of nine other soldiers were turned over to the U.S. authorities by communist forces. When his remains were handed over, no personal items of any kind were included with them, and the identity was listed as "unknown." U.S. government personnel performed a skeletal autopsy and confirmed Corporal Sanders's identification. He was identified by "favorable dental records, highly favorable physical profile, and proximity of his body to last known location." Also, the official report referred to a healed break in one of his foot bones. The records noted that "the proximal phalanx of the left second metatarsal had a healed break." The Sanders family stated that Corporal Sanders had never broken his toe and that it must not be his body in the casket. I explained to the family that, in the young, bone can heal very quickly. Corporal Sanders could have broken his toe at some point in his life and never realized it, never seeking medical aid. That break could have occurred before he ever left home, or he might have broken it on his tour of duty, simply ignoring the pain because of more pressing concerns. Still they wanted to know for certain.

The Sanders family requested my assistance in exhuming the body, providing a profile of the remains to see if it matched their loved one's description, and collecting a bone sample from the remains to send to a certified DNA laboratory. The family's ultimate disposition of the remains would depend on authentication of the identity or confirmation of their doubt. If indeed the remains were not those of Corporal Sanders, the military would then become involved. Once more I expressed concern about my participation. Shelley Belgard asked if I would just review the skeletal autopsy report before I gave them a definite no. Reluctantly, I agreed.

The army's report contained various bits of information about the recovered remains, including a dental chart outlining Corporal Sanders's dental work while in the army. Through multiple inquiries the Sanders family had learned that antemortem x-rays no longer existed. However, the precise written records noted dental fillings he had received, plus three tooth extractions. Those records could be used to help eliminate him as the person in the burial or confirm that the remains in the burial were his. I began to give the exhumation serious consideration, but we hit a slight snag in the discussions.

In this instance, "an interested party" contacted me and suggested that if the remains were not those of Corporal Sanders, the federal government might have moral and monetary culpability. My response was an immediate phone call to Shelley to advise her that I would not be involved in any case where there was the potential for suing the federal government. The September 11 attacks had already occurred, and I personally felt that the last thing anyone needed was to have to deal with a legal case in which many, if not all, of the principals were quite possibly dead. Though sympathetic to the Sanders family's request, I suggested that they find someone else to help them.

However, the family stated that suing anyone was the last thing they wanted to do. The "interested party" disappeared. But unfortunately, Corporal Sanders's mother died a short while later. I thought the whole thing would end there, but Lloyd Sanders called and explained how devastating it had been for his family all these years and how important it was to his mother's memory to pursue the issue. I felt reassured by his sincerity and once again began to consider helping them.

Quite frankly, the exhumation offered a number of possible benefits. Not only was it a chance for me to do something honorable to help the family of a soldier who had died for our country, it also represented a research opportunity with the potential for practical application. I have a strong interest in the degree of preservation of prehistoric, historic, and forensic burials in trying to understand postmortem interval and the impact of taphonomic, or weathering, processes on human remains. Though the prehistoric period offers its own unique challenges, historic and forensic situations vary somewhat according to the interpretation of those terms. Something is generally referred to as "historic" if it is at least a century old. In Louisiana, in legal terms, a body or set of remains is no longer "forensic" if it has been longer than fifty years since the person died. After that, it falls, somewhat prematurely, into the historic realm. Corporal Sanders's grave was just shy of fifty years old, and documenting the preservation of his remains, especially if intact DNA still existed in his bones or teeth, would provide valuable reference information for future forensic and recent historic cases in a burial context. I told Lloyd this up front, and he and his family were comfortable with my research interest. However, something completely out of our control presented a potential roadblock to any possibility of obtaining a positive identification of the remains through the use of DNA technology.

Following the Korean War, as part of Operation Glory, some soldiers' remains were first taken to the Kokura mortuary in Japan, where they were prepared for shipment to the United States if identified or transported to Hawaii to be buried in the Punchbowl National Cemetery there if unidentified. Today, it is estimated that hundreds of Americans remain unidentified at Punchbowl and thousands of others remain unaccounted for from the Korean War era. Shelley Belgard, as well as representatives from the U.S. Army's Central Identification Laboratory in Hawaii (called CILHI at the time), had noted that the remains that had gone through that mortuary had been covered with "some type of powder," perhaps a formalin (diluted formaldehyde) powder. It seems that the powder either destroyed the DNA altogether or inhibited its extraction and ultimate amplification. In the past, that mysterious powder had thwarted efforts to identify fragmented bones as belonging to specific individuals. On hearing this, I consulted with my friend and colleague Gwen Haugen, a forensic anthropologist at CILHI, and she confirmed it. She noted that in one case in particular, bones from that era appeared to be in pristine condition, looking as though the person had been dead for only a year or less. When their laboratory attempted to extract DNA, they came up empty handed. If that powder was present in Corporal Sanders's casket, we might hit a DNA dead end.

Once again, I discussed this with the Sanders family. They understood, but I think they had waited so long that they were desperate to try anything. We knew that the meticulous dental records prepared by the army could go a long way to help confirm or deny that the remains in the casket were those of Corporal Sanders. Finally, after more than a year of discussion, jumping through the legal hoops required for exhumation of a body, arranging the logistics for such a project, and mourning the death of their mother, the family was anxious to see it through to the end. I agreed to help.

That was what had brought me to the small country cemetery on that particular day in the summer of 2003. The original plan had been for us to take the remains back to the LSU FACES Lab in Baton Rouge, where we could examine them at our leisure for a few weeks. The more I thought about it, however, the more I felt that would not be necessary, since our main goal was a skeletal profile, a comparison of dental charts, and removal of bone and tooth samples for DNA analysis. I asked the Sanders family to see if they could find a laboratory where our team could examine the remains in an undisturbed setting for five or six hours of intensive analysis. If they could find such a place locally, the remains would not leave Arkansas, and they would not have to worry about what to do with the casket and an open grave until we could release the remains. Also, we would not have to worry over whether transport of potentially fragile remains might damage their integrity and affect our analysis. We were all relieved when a local funeral home director agreed to allow us to use his embalming laboratory for the analysis. Though not ideal, it would probably suffice.

My research associate Ginny Listi, graduate student Helen Bouzon, and I watched the backhoe operator work around the tombstones near Corporal Sanders's grave. I glanced to one side and saw the tombstone for his mother. Though she had not lived to see this day, the Sanders family believed their mother was at peace, and perhaps soon the rest of the family would be also. I knew that we would know something in a few hours.

The exhumation was scheduled to begin between 9:00 and 10:00 A.M. By that time, the members of the Sanders family had arrived, as well as a veteran from the Korean War and his wife. They had been introduced to the Sanders family through Shelley Belgard and wanted to be present to honor Corporal Sanders. Shelley said she knew of no other soldier from the Korean War who had been exhumed from his grave once returned and buried in the United States. To this day, I do not know if that is actually the case.

The backhoe began to get close to the casket. In my most diplomatic manner, I explained to the family that the casket could have leaked and that we might not have any remains with enough integrity for analysis. I stopped short of noting that exposure to the elements for almost fifty years could result in total destruction of the bones. I had seen it before, but I decided to hold off on any dire predictions until we actually saw the casket. Lynda, Corporal Sanders's sister, was the only person present at the cemetery in 2003 who remembered the details of her brother's funeral in 1955. I asked her if she could recall any specifics about her brother's casket. She was a teenager at the time, she said, and clearly remembered that he was buried in some type of "bronze-colored" casket. What we had just hit was not a bronze casket. It was, in fact, a metal vault, and it seemed eerily familiar. Once more, I asked Lynda if she recognized it. Neither she nor any other family member recalled any provision of a vault for Corporal Sanders. If the vault was still sealed, the casket might be also.

Slowly, the backhoe operator and the funeral home director raised the vault. Heavy bands held it securely as the operator moved it to an area away from the rest of the graves (FIGURE 3). The vault swung ever so slightly with the movement of the backhoe, and it became obvious why it had seemed so familiar. There was no mistaking its manufacturer. The tag on the side read "Clark," the same brand of vault in which the casket of Dr. Carl Austin Weiss, the alleged assassin of Huey Long, Louisiana's infamous governor, had been buried. "Guaranteed for Life" was Clark's motto. In Weiss's case, the sound Clark vault didn't help. When we exhumed his body in the early 1990s, after he had been buried for more than fifty years, the vault was preserved, but the wooden casket inside the vault was not. Though his soft tissue remains were partially intact, they

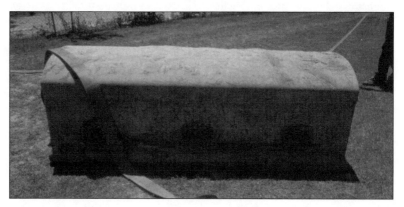

FIGURE 3.
Corporal Sanders's burial vault

had deteriorated beyond the point where the investigators could conduct the special analysis they hoped to perform. On the other hand, on this day in 2003, we were not dealing with soft tissue. Good bone preservation was our goal.

Lloyd and the volunteers worked for several minutes to loosen the bolts beneath the vault that held the top securely in place. Sweating profusely in the summer heat, they were finally able to do so. Excitedly, we watched as the vault cover was removed and the casket was revealed—all shiny and bronze, glistening in the sun. Lynda had remembered correctly. The casket looked new, its decorative florals, handles, escutcheons (screw covers), and other trim were perfectly preserved. Our hopes for good preservation of what rested inside the casket rose dramatically.

The men loaded the bronze casket onto the truck, and our motorcade made its way down the dirt road and back to town. I knew I would never see the cemetery again and hoped for positive results, especially for the sake of the mother whose remains now rested alongside an empty grave.

Knowing that our analysis could take hours, we decided to grab a quick lunch before we started our work. Experience had taught us not to tackle any case on an empty stomach. We ate lunch in almost complete silence as each of us was thinking of what lay ahead. As I had no idea what the remains would be like, old doubts began to sneak into my mind once more.

Finally, it was time. The funeral home director removed the screws that held the top of the casket in place. He popped the seal. Immediately, a very strong, pungent odor filled the room. It seemed foreign to me, a most unfamiliar, penetrating smell. Of course, it should not be from decay. According to the records, Corporal Sanders's remains were only bones. A slight hint of formalin was suggested, but, unlike formalin, which I had encountered on many occasions, this odor caused a strangely uncomfortable sensation in my nose and throat. The smell would persist throughout the entire analysis and would force us (even with masks in place) to take occasional breaks in the fresh air in order to get relief for our lungs. But at this preliminary phase, we were trying to decide if the odor came from a source we could identify. Was it the glue that was used to seal the casket? Was it something inside the casket itself? We could not tell, but at all times, we were careful not to breathe too deeply when we approached the casket. The air circulation in the funeral home's preparation laboratory helped little to ease the discomfort when the intensity of the odor increased as we lifted the casket's lid. All eyes on the casket, we leaned forward in anticipation.

Though I am sometimes surprised by things we encounter in our line of work, I was not prepared for what lay before me. Not only had Clark's vault remained sealed, but so had the casket. Lying on a bed of perfectly preserved, off-white cotton quilted pillows, which looked as though they had been placed there the day before, was what we refer to as a bundle burial (FIGURES 4 and 5). I gazed silently at the bundle, a little stunned, I must admit. Here was strong evidence—almost fifty years after the fact—that even in the past, we honored our fallen heroes. The care that had gone into the preparation and presentation of a set of skeletal remains placed in a casket that was presumed at the time would never be opened again was overwhelming.

An army green military blanket folded in a bundle, approximately three feet in length and containing the presumed remains, lay in the casket. Tied neatly with satin ribbons, it was wedged securely in place by several small rolls of canvas bags filled with what felt like sand. All ends of the blanket were tucked tightly with military precision and pinned together with large safety pins. Attached to one section of the bundle was a metal tag with Corporal Sanders's name and serial number on it.

I felt the scientist in me dissolving as strong emotions came quickly to the forefront. I didn't want to go any further. I didn't want to know if there were bones in the bundle. For one of the few times in my professional career, I wanted to leave the past in the past. What if inside the bundle was just more sand? What in the world would I do then? As comic relief for myself, I thought, "You have really stepped in it this time, girl." Quickly touching the top end of the blanket, I was reassured to feel a round object that seemed to be a skull. Intuitively, I knew at least that someone's remains rested in this casket.

I stepped away from the casket and motioned for Ginny to photo-

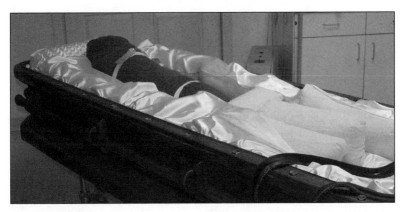

FIGURE 4.
Inside the casket

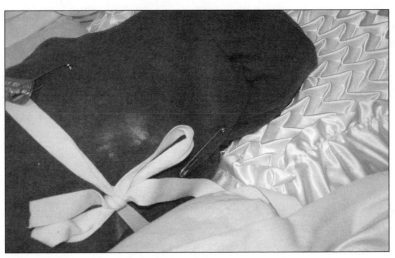

FIGURE 5.
Close-up of bundle burial

graph the bundle. Even if the remains turned out to be someone other than Corporal Sanders's, we had to document the care that had been provided for this person. For the Sanders family present that day and for many other soldiers' families who have had doubt about the treatment of the remains of their loved ones, this evidence was proof positive that somewhere on foreign soil almost a half century ago, our fallen heroes were prepared for their final rest in the respectful manner they so deserved.

Though we were momentarily slowed by the sight of the bundle, my great hope was that in a few moments we would be looking at the bones of Corporal Sanders. I could not imagine the family's disappointment if the remains were those of a stranger or, worse still, some foreign lad who had never heard of Arkansas, much less experienced the sun rising over a free horizon.

All of these crazy last-minute thoughts filled my mind as I slowly opened the thick, heavy blanket. When I removed the final pin and pulled back the last fold, once again everyone leaned in toward the casket. My eyes went immediately to the skull. "Young male," I thought, relieved. However, something else demanded my attention. Everywhere I looked, a powderlike material filled the blanket. It covered all the bones, including the skull, piles and piles of grayish white powder. "This must be the dreaded mortuary powder everyone has talked about," I thought to myself. I looked at the family and said, "This is just what we did not want to find, but let's work around it for now."

Once the family looked quickly at the bones, we asked that they wait outside while we completed our analysis. They of course understood.

Gently brushing the powder from the bones, we removed the bones from the blanket and laid them on the autopsy table in anatomical order. We then closed the casket to minimize the strong odor coming from it. Our preliminary idea that the odor might have been related to the glue used to seal the casket seemed accurate. By closing the casket, we greatly reduced the intensity of the smell. We knew that the odor was not coming from the powder that still clung to all of the bones.

Starting with the cranium, we carefully measured it and entered all measurements into our laptop computer, equipped with the software program FORDISC. That program, designed and developed at the University of Tennessee, assigns sex and race to a skull. Both Ginny and I measured the cranium independently and remeasured any site if our

individual results disagreed by more than two millimeters. FORDISC results indicated the skull was that of a male.

Race evaluation was a little more tenuous, but cranial features helped
us there. The dropped eye orbits, orthonathic lateral profile, and inter-
mediate nasal opening suggested it was the skull of a white male. The
skull also had a high cranial vault, moderate anterior nasal spine, and
pinched nasal root, all indicators of white ancestry. Finally, the interorbital breadth fit into Caucasoid, or white, parameters.

Next, we each completed a dental chart and once again compared one
to the other. Though we had Corporal Sanders's government records with
us, we did not have time to check for all consistencies. Generally speaking, however, they seemed to agree. We knew that when we returned to
our lab, we would study the records more closely. What we confirmed
immediately was that the extractions that Corporal Sanders had in the
military compared favorably with our preliminary examination of the remains. We would leave the final determination to Dr. Robert Barsley,
forensic odontologist, and our research partner for many years.

Our hands flew as we measured and remeasured all of the bones. The
preservation was impressive. The bones were as solid as any we might see
of a person who had been dead for no more than a year or so. Our friend
at CILHI had warned us of this unusual preservation, and the chill of her
dire prediction about the DNA had never left my mind. I only hoped
this case might be different.

Several hours passed, and our occasional breaks outside would find us
looking into the patient eyes of a family who wanted and needed some
information before we left Arkansas. Finally, we had done all that we
could do in a laboratory with no x-ray machine and limited tools. We
had assessed all bones and teeth and had measured everything we could
measure. We had encountered no foot bone that appeared to be broken,
but we had no way of knowing what the postmortem x-ray mentioned
in the government report had revealed about the broken bone. The break
was obviously slight but discernable in their x-ray image. Another important consideration was that the bone mentioned in the report may not

even have been Corporal Sanders's. We had to remember that various persons' bones may have been commingled in the remains returned by the communists.

Our last task was to take a bone and tooth sample for DNA analysis. One of the most troubling things for physical anthropologists is accidental damage to a bone or teeth. To sample a skeleton for DNA, however, damage is done deliberately. DNA technology, while arguably one of the most important scientific advances of modern times, required that we cut out at least one section of bone and extract one tooth. We did so.

Before we placed the remains back inside the casket, we also took a sample of the peculiar powder. Gwen had told me that CILHI had already analyzed the powder, but we were anxious to have someone else take a look, too.

Our team stepped out into the hot air on that late summer afternoon and I spoke to the family. "We have the remains of a young male, probably white, whose skeletal and dental profile compare favorably with the antemortem dental records for your brother," I told them. "He may well be your brother, but we will wait until confirmation of the consistency of the dental charts and results of the DNA analysis."

As we knew they would be, Lloyd and his family were very grateful for our help. I knew they were not quite convinced that the young man in the bronze casket was their beloved brother, but they could be content to wait a while longer to hear what the DNA laboratory reported. On the other hand, they planned to rebury the remains early the next morning where they came from, near the grave of their mother.

We piled into our truck and headed home. The six-hour drive, much like the marathon analysis, would be completed mostly in silence. We were exhausted, pleased, and still a little tentative. The physical and mental stress had taken its toll.

The first phone call I made from my office the next work day was to Dr. Frank Fronzek, an LSU chemist. Frank had helped me on a historical case before, and I knew he would relish another challenge. He dropped by the next day, heard the story, and took a small sample of the powder. Also that day, Ginny hand-carried the DNA samples to the ReliaGene laboratory in New Orleans. The wait for the results would be a lot longer than we had imagined.

Frank's results came first. "Mary," he said, "you have what is a mixture of several different rocks that have been ground into a fine powder. There is calcite and gypsum, which may have acted as dehydrating powder to prevent molding or even to reduce any odor associated with the remains."

"What could this do to DNA?" I asked.

"What do you mean?"

I told him the story of CILHI's results. "Interesting," was his only comment.

A few weeks later, I contacted Wanda LeBlanc, a chemist down the hall from me in the geology department. Since Wanda worked with geologists, I thought she might have a different perspective on the powder, though rocks are rocks. Wanda graciously agreed to place some of the powder in her x-ray diffractometer to "cook" overnight and see what it said. The diffractometer registered high percentages of calcite and gypsum, identical to Frank's findings. These minerals are found in Drierite, a desiccant, Wanda said. The powder's constituents had been confirmed by two scientists. Most likely, it had been placed on the remains to dry them out and/or diminish odor. That protocol obviously was followed in all cases, regardless of whether soft tissue was present. I had a bad feeling that the powder may have worked too well.

For the results of the DNA analysis, the Sanders family waited six months before hearing from ReliaGene analyst Gina Pineda. Gina noted that she had tried every extraction process known to exist and consistently was unable to extract DNA from the bone or the tooth. True to the experience of others, no DNA was forthcoming. Lloyd and his family accepted ReliaGene's results with good spirits. I told them that Dr. Barsley felt comfortable that the postmortem dental records we made compared favorably with Corporal Sanders's antemortem records. Only antemortem and postmortem x-rays, evidence we did not have, could truly confirm a positive identification. However, Dr. Barsley noted the odds were that Corporal Sanders's extractions and fillings had not been duplicated in someone else's teeth. The odds against someone other than Corporal Sanders with identical dental details being present in exactly that place in the world at precisely that moment in history would have been even greater. Dr. Barsley said he believed the remains in the casket were those of Corporal James B. Sanders. We agreed.

4

Friends for Life

THE small beagle who raced ahead of his owner along the bayou
that day stopped abruptly, sniffing something in the loose soil
just a few feet from the water's edge. He began to dig vigorously
as his owner approached the area. The odor was so powerful that the
owner noticed it, too, the unmistakable smell of death.

By the time the man reached his dog, a portion of a decaying body
was protruding from the soil. Almost gagging on the stench and the real-
ization of what he was witnessing, the owner quickly leashed his dog and
ran toward his truck, signaling the beginning of a case that would con-
sume detectives, prosecutors, defense attorneys, and me for years to
come.

Kim Kolomb, a forensic investigator with the Louisiana State Police
Crime Laboratory, called that day. "Mary," she said, "there's a decom-
posed body that's been found in a shallow grave down south of Baton
Rouge along a bayou. Could you look at the body and at the grave? The
forensic entomologists have already been there." Of course, I agreed. Kim
and I had been working on cases together for years, and I had been con-
sulting for the crime lab since I started graduate school in 1981. She had a
most uncommon instinct about such cases and more often than not was
right on target.

I met Kim at the crime lab, and we headed south. First, we stopped
by the parish morgue in the little town and reviewed the remains. The
body was in an advanced stage of decomposition, as are many of our
cases, and, later, the autopsy would add to its disarray. The skull was
highly fragmented, and decaying tissue obscured much of what was obvi-

ously dramatic trauma to the bone. Kim explained that the coroner's autopsy would take place that day, but after that, she would really like for me to examine the body. I told her I would be glad to review the case and give my opinion. Forensic anthropologists are invited in on cases by the agencies involved. Generally speaking, in a coroner's system such as the one in Louisiana, we do not have legal standing that automatically requires our involvement in a case. In states that have a medical examiner's system, some medical examiners have an anthropologist on call and routinely consult with the forensic anthropologist on many cases, especially if skeletal trauma is involved. In the last twenty-five years, coroners in Louisiana have become well acquainted with our work and often do consult with us. When Kim related to the sheriff and coroner's representatives that she thought it would be a good idea for me to examine the body, they readily agreed. They also agreed to transport the body to my lab at LSU after autopsy.

Once we arrived at the bayou, we followed the well-beaten path to the shallow grave where the body had been found. We went to work immediately, discovering only a little body residue that had been left behind by the first recovery team. As most are, they, too, probably were anxious to get relief from the overwhelming stench of a decomposing body in Louisiana's summer heat, but their comprehensive recovery effort had missed nothing significant. When I was satisfied that no other human remains were left in the soil, we turned our attention to the burial pit itself.

No more than eighteen inches at its greatest depth, the pit offered evidence of a truism about most killers: they're lazy. Whoever had placed the body in the grave obviously had dug the hole very quickly, probably in a hurry to dispose of it, totally oblivious to how quickly a decomposing body can be discovered. We described and measured the pit for future reference. Occasionally, digging instruments, especially shovels, can leave tool marks in the wall of the burial pit, which can help lead authorities to the very tool that was used to dig the hole. Also, depth and appearance of a burial pit, especially a deep one, can suggest the element of premeditation. Someone who plans such a crime in advance might take the time to dig a hole deep enough to reduce the chance of immediate discovery.

While we measured the pit, a helicopter overhead signaled the inevitable approach of news reporters who had heard about the case. As hard as it was to believe, they landed nearby and I heard them noisily calling out to one another as they made their way down the winding trail to the bayou. Appearing almost out of nowhere, a young, polished female reporter in a flowing dress and beige high heels approached us.

I rocked back on my heels and almost laughed out loud as she asked, "Is it okay to stand right here?" Her question came as she simultaneously stepped in an area immediately adjacent to the burial pit where we had just deposited some body residue. I couldn't help but smile inwardly at the knowledge of one pair of good-looking pumps being dumped unceremoniously into the first available garbage can once she realized the unmistakable odor of death was not just up her nose. The reporters stayed only briefly. The real news soon would be on its way to my lab, and public interest would wither and die before the case was closed years later.

The body was obviously that of a young man, and the pathologist concluded that he had died of a single gunshot wound to the head. Authorities felt they might know the victim's identity. A young man from out of state had been working in south Louisiana when he was reported missing almost two weeks prior to the discovery of the body. Alarmed that they had not heard from their loved one, the family had called the local sheriff's office to ask for help. After the hunter discovered the body, Dr. Lamar Meek and Ms. Jeanine Tessmer, the entomologists who were called to the scene, gave their opinion. Later, they noted that the fly activity fit well into the time line of the young man's disappearance. Once the flies located the body (a matter of a few minutes if the soil was loose enough for them to detect the body and get to any part of it), they laid their eggs immediately. Those eggs hatched in eight to twelve hours. In two weeks or less, the flies' larvae had gone through their entire life cycle and finally emerged as adult flies. As a matter of fact, we saw many flies hanging on nearby bushes. When they first emerge from the pupae, which look like small, brown beans, flies are helpless and have to "season" or "cure" their wings through a drying process before they can fly anywhere. Such flies that are just hanging out on nearby bushes at a death scene are great indicators of the minimum amount of time elapsed since other flies laid their eggs, or oviposited, on a body.

The stage of decomposition of the body fit also, though the shallow burial had slowed the process to a minor degree. A general rule of thumb is that it will take at least three to four times as long for a buried body to decompose as it will for a body on the surface. My experience has been that some buried bodies can retain soft tissue for many, many years. It's related in part to how deep the body is buried and what type of covering is placed over the body. This shallow burial delayed the decomposition process only slightly, probably because some animal had loosened the soil around it and allowed the flies to get to it. We finished our descriptions and drawings and walked back toward our vehicles. The real work had not yet begun.

By the time I received the body in my lab, dental x-rays provided by the family were already on their way, and in just a brief period Dr. Barsley and I identified him. Jeremy Brown was a twenty-three-year-old white male who had come to south Louisiana to earn extra money when he could not find work in his home state. His car was found later, abandoned in an adjacent state. After positive identification of his body, his family was anxious to have the remains returned. In fact, they wanted to cremate him.

Once a coroner releases the remains, a family has every right to handle the disposition of its loved one's body as it sees fit. As an advocate for the victim, especially in criminal cases, I cringe at the word "cremate." I discourage it in every instance, especially if evidence of violence is present on the skeleton. That is one of the most important reasons for a forensic anthropologist to examine a person's remains. Evidence of trauma great enough to damage bones suggests considerable violence being perpetrated against the individual. My analysis of Jeremy's remains would include strong evidence of such violence. In his case, though he had been identified, the coroner had not yet released his body because I had not finished my work.

In my laboratory, I removed the decaying tissue from Jeremy's skull and glued the skull back together again. Extensive trauma was apparent. Instead of just a single gunshot wound near the top of his head on the right-hand side, as the pathologist had concluded, putrefactive tissue had hidden a similar injury just behind his earhole on the same side of the skull. The fracture patterns confirmed that the first injury was the one on the top of the skull. The fracture lines radiating out from the second bullet hole behind his ear stopped when they reached the fracture lines made by the first bullet. Just like the fracture patterns in a vehicle's windshield, subsequent fractures do not cross the line of first damage.

So what? one might ask. He was shot twice in the head instead of once. He still died from gunshot wounds to the head. This finding did not alter the determination of death made by the pathologist. While that was true, I had not completed my analysis. Approximately two centimeters forward from the bullet hole on the top of his skull was an entirely different type of trauma. Rather than the presence of jagged, discreet pieces of skull often associated with a high-velocity trauma (where the skull can be reconstructed like a puzzle), a small perimortem injury with a different appearance altogether was obvious in the bone. Blunt-force trauma of some kind had forced the bone inward toward the brain. That was not a bullet wound. Something had hit the head and had hit it hard. The location of the injury immediately adjacent to the fracture lines produced by the first bullet was also telling. Only one edge of the two primary fracture lines caused by high-velocity trauma was damaged by blunt force. This suggested that the fractures caused by the bullet had occurred prior to the blunt-force injury.

As I examined the postcranial remains (those below the skull), I found blunt-force trauma on several ribs on the right-hand side of the body and on the upper right arm. The ribs were broken in halves by blunt force, and the humerus had a small hole about the size of a pencil eraser punched inward into the shaft near the shoulder. This injury aligned with the injuries to the ribs and suggested that some type of blunt-force trauma had also occurred on the right-hand side of Jeremy's upper chest region. Clearly, those were not bullet injuries. The young man had been shot and also had been beaten. I called the sheriff's office, and they informed me that two suspects had been arrested and one was talking. The details of his story would make even a hardened criminal cringe at what the two suspects had done to their "friend."

It seems that the two had only met Jeremy a few weeks earlier and had become fast friends as they worked together. Weekly paychecks had been passed out when the two men suggested to Jeremy that they take his gun for target practice down on the bayou. The story goes that the pair stopped at a hardware store and bought a shovel before meeting Jeremy for a couple of drinks at a local night club. They left the club and headed to the bayou. At the target practice site, they took turns shooting Jeremy's gun; then one of them turned it on him.

Even more chilling were additional details that were revealed when the shooter confessed to the sheriff's detectives that he indeed was the shooter. When Jeremy did not die immediately from the gunshots, one of the two perpetrators took the shovel and hit Jeremy over the head with it. Finally, Jeremy died. For the sum of twelve hundred dollars, split two ways, they killed him.

Jeremy's family was still anxious to put the tragedy behind them and requested that Jeremy's remains be sent to the crematorium. I strongly recommended that the damaged bones be retained for future reference, especially since the second suspect disputed having anything at all to do with Jeremy's death, saying that he was unsure about what happened.

We were allowed to retain the damaged bones, and the defense attorneys for the accused man who denied participation in the murder visited my laboratory to discuss the remains. They asked me if I knew that cows grazed in the area where Jeremy was found. I seemed to recall seeing cow patties, but I had not given it much thought. One of the attorneys informed me that he could argue in court that the damage I saw as blunt force could have occurred from a cow stepping on Jeremy's head in the shallow grave. I responded by noting that had that occurred, the injury would not have been so isolated and the fracture pattern would have been much more widespread based on the size and shape of the average cow's hoof. I told him that in my opinion the instrument that caused the injury to the skull and to the arm had some configuration quite different from a cow's hoof.

Over the next few months, the defense attorneys requested that the court allow them to get opinions from other forensic anthropologists. The court agreed, and Jeremy's injuries were reviewed by three other forensic anthropologists. One, whom the defense attorneys brought from out of state to review the case in my laboratory, eventually noted in his report that the injury I highlighted as being separate from the bullet wounds was indeed caused by blunt force. The other two out-of-state forensic anthropologists agreed also: high-velocity and blunt-force trauma to the skull. Later, I was told that at least one of the anthropologists noted that the shape of the injury on the skull exactly matched the curl at the top of the shovel's blade. I had never seen the shovel.

In the end, this was a case in which a young man was trusting of new friends he had met on a new job. However, they were just acquaintances who were filled with such greed and malice in their hearts that it meant nothing to them to strike down a fellow human being before he reached the age of twenty-five. His bones revealed the true story of what happened to him just prior to his death, and eventually the people who committed the crime were given life in prison without benefit of parole. Ironically, one of them, not much older than Jeremy, has already died in prison.

5

Sisters

THOUSANDS and thousands of vehicles traveled the overpass ramp every day. Unknown to the drivers, something lay beneath it, waiting to be discovered. For two years, the remains rested there until a lone armadillo pawed at the loose soil, exposing a rounded, human skull.

The structural engineer pulled the metal grate from the small opening and waved his powerful flashlight inside—something scurried in one corner and caught his attention—the sleepy-eyed armadillo. It sat next to what the engineer first thought to be another armadillo—he looked a little closer, and closer still. A human skull stared back at him from the recesses of the overpass ramp as cars could be heard thundering down the ramp overhead. For a moment, he thought he was mistaken. However, what had begun as a routine inspection to confirm the structural integrity of the overpass ramp would end in a tale that would touch even the most jaded of hearts.

It seems like yesterday, though years have passed since I was called to the center of one of Louisiana's bustling cities to help recover the remains of a body that had been found accidentally. When my phone rang that day, the coroner's investigator on the other end spoke in rapid fire. "Mary, we need your help. Can you come immediately? Someone found a human skull sticking out of some dirt in the crawl space beneath a concrete ramp. A person must be buried there." He didn't have to say anymore.

"I'm on my way," I replied. At that time in my career, I still drove my own vehicle to scenes and did not have the luxury of graduate assistants to help. I knew that if the body had to be transported to my laboratory, the agency involved could take care of that unless it was just bones. Many a set of bones had made their way to my lab in my well-used minivan.

When I arrived at the scene, it was crawling with detectives, policemen, and coroner's investigators. Heading toward the ramp, I noticed that it was totally enclosed in concrete except for the small opening through which the structural engineer had crawled. I got down on my hands and knees and peeked in. The air was stale and musty. Gingerly, I crawled in and remained on all fours because I could not stand. At five foot two, I'm not the tallest anthropologist standing, but even I had to bend over to clear the ceiling of the interior of the ramp.

Shadows cast by the lights that had been strung inside the dank enclosure danced along the walls in eerie shapes. The lead investigator pointed to the skull uncovered by the armadillo. From what I could see, it looked quite small, perhaps a female or a teenager. A relatively large pile of dirt covered what might be the rest of a body. The investigators had done well. I was sure that they had been tempted to go ahead and uncover everything but chose to wait for me. I thanked them for their patience.

On the other side of the pile of dirt, which was approximately six feet long and nearly three feet wide, was a fairly large hole. It was apparent that the perpetrator had dug the hole and used it as what we call a "borrow pit" for dirt to cover the body. On multiple occasions in the past we had shown that killers were lazy. This seemed to exemplify another truism about them: they can also be very stupid. If whoever had done this had simply dug a little deeper and placed the body in the hole, rather than leaving it on top of the ground, it might never have been discovered. Though I didn't have time to dwell on it, I knew that we were not dealing with an Einstein.

I quickly assessed the situation and we went to work. It had already gotten dark outside, and it was suffocating inside; we needed to get the body out. Yet my archaeological training had taught me that haste makes waste and, as we say in archaeology, "When you recover the past, you destroy it at the same time." This certainly applies to a death scene. You can never put it back the way it was. Better do it right the first time. The fact that the surroundings were uncomfortable for us was not a consideration.

Taking a closer look at what I could see of the skull, I motioned for the investigators to work around the shoulder region while I whisked away the loose soil from the exposed bone to get a better view. Once I had done that, I realized that the skull was most likely that of a female, black, and very young, probably a teenager. Her cranial joints, or sutures, were still wide open. Most of the cranial joints fuse when a person is in her mid to late twenties or even later. I stopped short of uncovering the skull completely and decided to move to the foot region, where we had noticed a girl's tennis shoe not far from the end of the dirt pile, close to the ramp's access window. It had to be related. I ignored the shoe but knew that I would have to come back to it before the night was over.

As the investigators continued to slowly clear away the soil around the shoulder region, I began to remove dirt from the area where I should find the legs and feet. I gently brushed away the soil until I uncovered a left tibia and fibula, the lower leg bones. Continuing to work in that area, I found the tibia and fibula from the opposite side. No clothing covered the legs. I could tell by the unfused long bones that we were probably looking at the remains of a young teenager. The ends of the femora and tibiae at the knee region were unfused, suggesting someone under eighteen years of age.

Then, as I was cleaning away a little more dirt, I struck a bone that should not have been there, another tibia, then another, then two fibulae. Four tibiae and four fibulae in all. I realized that we were working on not just one set of remains but two. The second was even smaller and younger than the first. I felt a sudden chill; not just one but two children lay in this makeshift tomb. I suppressed the urge to scream my anger out loud. I was restrained only in part by how it would have looked to the investigators, as I knew my voice would reverberate off the walls with a chilling cacophony. (I had not been given a role in the senior play in high school based on my acting talent. My teacher had suggested at the time that my voice could easily be heard in the next parish over.)

Moving back to the area where the skull rested, I carefully began to clean around it. It was getting late; we needed some answers and we needed them fast. Once more, the loose soil was a blessing. Within an hour, we had uncovered another skull and the rest of the two small bodies. They were completely skeletonized, obviously having been there at least six months to a year or more.

One of the detectives crawled over to a corner of the ramp's interior and found a plastic bag. Opening it, he discovered a few bits and pieces of paper and a pair of girl's gym shorts. The name of a school was imprinted on the shorts. A lightbulb came on in his head; he remembered that two young black children had been reported missing months earlier. Their home life was such that authorities had encountered them when they had tried to run away before. When they were reported missing a second time, everyone thought they had done the same thing again. The detective quickly crawled from under the ramp, ran to his car, and called headquarters, asking for detailed descriptions of the missing girls. I knew he had hit the mark. They were the ones. I didn't need the description to tell me that.

We finished uncovering the remains and documented everything we saw. The drawing and photographs would attest to the awful truth: two small children were placed almost on top of one another on the ground's surface and covered with dirt dug from a hole immediately adjacent to their bodies.

We finally crawled from under the ramp that night exhausted and angry at whoever had committed this despicable crime. I carefully placed the remains in my vehicle to transport them to my laboratory for analysis. My day's work was almost over. I drove back to Baton Rouge with a heavy heart. Some days I absolutely hated my job; that was one of those days.

The next day I began to evaluate the skeletal remains. One of the two children was probably between ten and twelve years of age, judging from dental development and fusion of the hipbones. The second molars in the dental arcade had recently erupted. That generally occurs between ten and twelve years of age, though it may happen earlier or be delayed. X-rays of the teeth showed that the second molars were fully developed. Also, each of the hipbones for that individual was still in two pieces. Though a hipbone starts out as three bones, the ilium and the ischium fuse together prior to puberty. Then the pubic bone fuses to those two bones during puberty.

The older child was most likely a female. Though sex is difficult to assess in children, her skeletal development was beyond that of the first child. The hipbones are the best bones in the skeleton for determining sex, and her hipbones were developed enough to indicate that she was female. She had a wide sciatic notch, a long pubic bone, and a concave sub-pubic angle, all female indicators.

The fusion of her hipbones was more advanced than the first child's; the three segments of each of her hipbones had fused into one bone. Her dental development also corresponded to that of a teenager. Her third molars, or wisdom teeth, were apparent in her x-rays and were at a developmental stage beyond that of the other child, though the roots of those teeth had not completed their growth. The roots of the third molars have usually completed their growth at around eighteen years of age. She clearly was younger than that.

A few days later, the investigators called with the news that no dental records existed for the two missing females. I was not surprised. They both had perfect teeth. DNA identification was not an option at that time. Instead, we decided to employ a technique that had had some success in the few cases in which it had been used, photographic superimposition. This technique requires that you have a good straight-forward photo of the person you are trying to identify. Using cameras and monitors, you then superimpose the skull over the photograph to determine if the shape of the skull fits the photo. The only drawback was that two of the top practitioners of the technique were at the Federal Bureau of Investigation and the Museum of Natural History at the Smithsonian Institution in Washington, D.C. Anxious to resolve this case, the sheriff approved the trip to Washington. Eileen Barrow, FACES Lab imaging specialist, and case detectives hopped a plane to Washington immediately. For hours, they tried to match up the photograph and the skull. In the end they were not comfortable with providing a positive identification. Eileen returned with the disappointing news.

I wanted to try something else. Drs. Barsley and Carr had come through before when we needed their expertise in odontology, and the fact that they had identified hundreds of people based on dental morphology was even more comforting. We decided to try the technique of superimposition once more at the LSU Dental School in New Orleans and focus on the shape of the teeth only. After hours of lining up the photograph with the skull of the older child in the region of the mouth and pinpointing all of the similarities in the shape of the anterior teeth, the odontologists agreed that, indeed, the teeth of the older victim matched those in the photo. One of the victims clearly was the older child who was thought to have run away. Though a smiling photo of the second child did not expose teeth, by virtue of known association and blood ties, physical attributes, and clothing, the second child was declared to be the younger sibling.

Once the identification was made, the detectives could concentrate on finding out who had committed this crime. Eventually, authorities had a suspect. However, in the end, they were never able to bring charges against him for the deaths of the two children. Ironically, a couple of years later, he received an extensive prison term for an unrelated crime.

I've often thought about those two children over the years; children's cases never leave you completely. Sometimes, I relive their images in my head, not the smiling faces in their photographs, but the ones I saw under the ramp. Though their skeletons helped us to identify them, they provided no clues as to what happened to them in their last few moments of life. I submit that the system happened to them. Their cries for help throughout their brief years—and it seems there were some—went unheeded. We failed them. We all failed them. We rushed to identify them after they were found dead, but we did not rush to save them while they were alive.

As a society, reportedly the greatest in the world, we allowed them to fall through the cracks. At the very least, we owed them a chance to grow up in an atmosphere without fear. All they ever wanted was a chance.

6

Alone in the Woods

A N unretrieved backpack was the only evidence that Peggy Watson had walked that way on that particular day. Sometimes Peggy would skip school, like any teenager, leaving her backpack behind a small bush at the edge of the school grounds to retrieve at the end of the day. But that day she never returned for the backpack. Her homecoming would be a most painful and long-awaited day for her family some eight years later.

The call came late one afternoon. The chief of detectives in a western Louisiana parish had a bone he wanted me to see. He asked, "Can I bring it to you, Mary?" He thought it was human but he wanted to be sure. In fact, he thought it was part of a human skull. His real interest lay in its close proximity to a tennis shoe that had been found not too far away from the bone—a girl's tennis shoe.

"Where did you find these?" I asked.

"Deep in the piney woods," he answered.

He arrived at my office early the next morning. Clean shaven, tall and lanky, he spoke with that polite southern voice that showed his mama had raised him right. He's one of a dying breed. He had spent his entire life in the small town where missing kids were those who just stayed out a little past their curfew. But there was one case, eights years ago, he said, that just tore out the hearts of those who lived in the close-knit community.

He told me the story of Peggy Watson and how she sometimes took a break from school but always returned at the end of the day. But on that day eight years before, she did not return. Volunteers searched the nearby

woods for weeks, knowing that she would not willingly have gone anywhere with a stranger. She was never found.

The detective broke the evidence tape on a brown paper bag and pulled
out the fragment of bone. I felt an adrenalin rush. Indeed, it was part of a
human skull, the calotte, or skullcap. It was small, what we call gracile,
with just the beginning of a nice, straight forehead. The parietals, the
bones on either side of the skull, were flared just a little, a characteristic
that females retain from infancy. Males do not. The sagittal suture, the
joint running down the middle of the skull, was wide open, or unfused,
supporting my assessment that it belonged to a person under twenty
years of age. I told the detective that he had the skullcap of a young
human, probably a teenager, and possibly female. The color of the bone
provided me with other clues. It was weathered gray, and the outer, or
cortical, bone was beginning to crack, or craze. I knew from past experience in Louisiana that such coloring and dryness were often associated
with skeletal remains that had been exposed to the elements for five to
ten years.

"What about the tennis shoe?" I asked him, though I knew it might
have nothing at all to do with the bone fragment. He pulled it from another bag. It was an unusual brand and had fared somewhat better than
the bone, though it, too, had some age on it. He told me the story of the
shoe. The teenager had been wearing shoes just like that one when she
disappeared. They were new at the time, and her mother had kept the
box they came in for eight long years.

"Will you help us search some more, Mary," he asked, "to see if we
can find anything that could be used to positively identify her or show
that this skull bone does not belong to her?" He had me hooked after he
had first said "tennis shoe" and "mother." I knew, however, that the odds
were not good after eight years. Also, the damage to the skullcap sup-
ported the assumption that animals had probably already destroyed the
other remains. Typically in cases where remains are found in the woods,
animals will leave the skull for the very last because it's hard for them to
get a good grip on, even with long canine teeth. Since this one was

mostly destroyed, I knew there would not be much more of the skeleton out there unless it had been protected somehow. Still, we had to try. We could attempt to extract DNA from the skullcap, but it was not the best bone to use for DNA identification. Positive identifications through the use of nuclear DNA were being done at the time, but the skull fragment might only have mitochondrial DNA, which was still in its infancy as an identification tool.

We made arrangements to meet the next morning. Before we parted, the detective asked if I thought a cadaver dog might help. I answered him truthfully. In the twenty-five or more of my cases where we had used cadaver dogs, especially when looking for completely skeletonized remains, our success rate had been less than good. However, we should try it if he wanted to do so. A friend of mine had a dog she was training. I called her and she agreed to go. She brought Sacket with her.

After a three-hour drive, we arrived at the road that was nearest the area where the bone had been found. We immediately began to search. Since it was fall, the light-colored bones should be fairly easy to see among the leaves. Unfortunately, they might also be covered by the leaves. Within five minutes, my sometimes good luck held. I found a significant portion of a left femur, the thighbone. It was small and gray, just like the skullcap. Clearly, it was human, and it was most likely part of the same skeleton. Unfortunately, that was the only thing we found the entire day. Earlier, the detective had shown me the place where the skullcap had been discovered. I dug around in that area with a trowel for several minutes but found nothing, my first mistake that day. In fact, I assumed that the skullcap had been carried into that area by some animal. Since the face was missing, the teeth may have long since been lost.

We covered thousands of square feet of land in the area where the shoe and the skullcap were found, but we ended up empty handed after finding that one piece of thighbone. At the end of the day we were exhausted, and the cadaver dog, Sacket, was lost. My second mistake of the day. His owner was getting a little nervous by the time we started packing up, but finally Sacket came wandering back just as we were about to leave.

I was disappointed that we had found nothing that could help us. So was the chief deputy, but our good luck was not over. He called me a couple of days later, very excited. He and his assistant had gone back to the site near where the skullcap had been found and had dug around in the soil a little more diligently than I had done. He found two teeth near where the calotte was found. I was excited for him but aggravated at myself for not finding them earlier. It didn't really matter, however. What did matter was now that we had the teeth, we could get Peggy's dental records and see if those particular teeth were present in the x-rays. If they were, we might know in a short time if the remains were Peggy's.

Nothing is ever as easy as we expect. Though it was known that Peggy had x-rays of her teeth, they were not found in a preliminary search. In reality, that is not so unusual. X-rays are sometimes lost, often destroyed after a certain period of time, and can even be misfiled within a lab's storage area. But Peggy's x-rays were never found.

We had one alternative. We could take the teeth, which are wonderful repositories for DNA, and have them analyzed at the ReliaGene laboratories in New Orleans. At the time, ReliaGene was one of the few certified DNA labs in the country that could perform such an analysis. I explained to the detective, however, that these tests would destroy the teeth. He understood, but he asked if I thought DNA would still be there after so long in the shallow soil. First of all, we really did not know how long they had been in the dirt. They may have fallen from the dental arcade only recently. If so, the bone could have protected them all those years. Additionally, one of my graduate students had just completed her thesis research on the preservation of mitochondrial DNA in bone that had been exposed to the natural elements in Louisiana. Her results were quite promising and showed that bone on the ground's surface in Louisiana for more than a decade still contained extractable DNA. Besides, we had already x-rayed the two teeth in every position we thought possible in case antemortem x-rays were located. Therefore, we felt comfortable that the teeth themselves could be put to far better use by trying to get DNA from them. The detective agreed, and so did Peggy's family.

Once again, ReliaGene proved how good they were. Not only did the teeth have DNA, it was easily matched to samples taken from Peggy's mom and dad. After eight long years, they could bury their daughter. The few pieces of bone and teeth we had for Peggy told the story of who she was. For the family, the sorrow of that reality would only subside with time. Eventually, they could go on with their lives knowing at least that their child had been found. We uncovered no evidence of what had happened to Peggy. The pain of not knowing exactly what had happened to their daughter would probably never leave them. Parents are not supposed to survive their children. The natural order was broken, and so were their hearts. Whoever committed this unspeakable crime has never been discovered.

They Walk Among Us

MANY strange cases have made their way to my laboratory over the years. Some are a little stranger than others. In the fall of 2001 I received a rather unusual phone call just before my morning class one day. The detective on the other end of the line sounded patient and experienced but a little concerned. "Miss Mary," he said, "I've got a situation I need a little help with."

After that, his story quickly entered the category "only in Louisiana," which I reserve for cases that defy logic and whose participants are surely candidates for the Darwin Awards (given, the awards' Web site says, to "salute the improvement of the human genome by honoring those who accidentally kill themselves in really stupid ways").

A hunter had called the sheriff's office the day before and relayed his tale. He was walking in the deep woods, he told the detective, and had headed toward a little creek bed he knew very well to see if any deer tracks could point him toward the prize buck that he always thought was just around the bend. The squirrels and blue jays were not about their usual business of chattering and squawking over territorial boundaries. In fact, he noted, an unusual calm had spread all across the forest as he quietly made his way down to the creek bed. He peered cautiously around two small yaupon hedges for a quick look-see into the dry creek. It was then that he saw it, immediately adjacent to hoofprints made by a deer that had traveled that way recently: another print in the soil—a large print, a very large print, more than a foot long and five or six inches wide, made by a manlike creature that had traveled that way about the same time as the deer. "Manlike creature" was a good description, the hunter continued, but it was not man. It had only four toes, four very large toes. Also, something on a nearby bush caught the light of the morning sun and glistened black against the fall foliage: hairs, long, black hairs, not human hairs. The hunter touched nothing but marked the spot, quickly retreated from the forest, and drove his truck to the nearest phone to call the sheriff's office. "Bigfoot is in Kisatchie Forest," he told the dispatcher.

"Yeah, sure," the dispatcher replied, "and Chicken Little says the sky is falling."

"Please come," the hunter yelled.

The sheriff's detective who got the case knew that he had better check it out because he figured the hunter had not called just the sheriff's office. By the time the detective and crime scene personnel neared the location described by the hunter, clouds of dust were billowing everywhere. Obviously, the hunter had told his friends.

The detective knew he had to do something because he had been raised with these guys and they were as trigger-happy as they come. He worried that they would end up shooting each other. He explained to me that he had gone to the site, made an impression of the footprint (FIG- URE 6), and collected the hairs. Could I give him an opinion on the hairs and footprint?

"Sure," I told him, "but Bigfoot is clearly out of my area of expertise." He laughed, probably for the first time that day.

"Miss Mary," he said, "I know it's not Bigfoot. I just need some science to show these locals. Why, I've had calls from all across the country already. National news people are on their way down here right now. It's a zoo, I tell you. So what do you need?"

"I need the hairs and I need to see the footprint."

"That reminds me," he said. "The footprint was right next to a big log, and the print was only an inch or two deep."

"Go on," I said, noting only a short pause in his thoughts.

"A few feet away were fresh deer tracks. They sank down in that creek bed at least three or more inches."

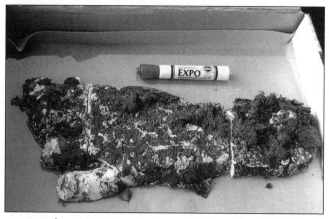

FIGURE 6.
Footprint cast of "Bigfoot"

"Are you trying to tell me that Bigfoot is very light on his feet?" He laughed again.

"Something like that," he chuckled. He got to my office within a couple of hours. I would love to have seen his speedometer reading.

I looked at the cast and said, "Yeah, that's a footprint, all right."

"What do you think about the four toes?"

"Well," I replied, "there's four of them."

"Yeah," he answered, "and some hotshot Sasquatch expert from Oregon says that any kind of bigfoot has to have five toes, like humans."

"So what you're saying then is that we have a bigfoot wannabe here?" I loved making that man laugh.

We took photographs of the cast, kept the hairs, and sent the detective home. I immediately contacted Cindy Henk in the electron microscopy lab. "Cindy, how would you like to make national news?" I asked her.

"Not particularly interested," she said. I told her the story, and she said to bring the hairs on over and she would use the scanning electron microscope (SEM) to get a close-up on them. I met her at the lab, and we sat down together as she opened the tube and placed them inside. Focusing on one of the hairs, she could easily distinguish its shape, its coarseness, its outer coating, and its ends (FIGURE 7). The SEM revealed

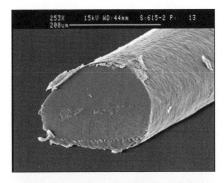

FIGURE 7.
"Bigfoot" hair, straight edge

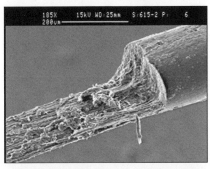

FIGURE 8.
"Bigfoot" hair, shaved edge

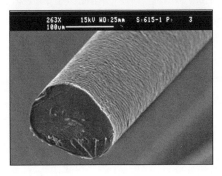

FIGURE 9.
Horse hair

a straight edge on one end and on the other end a straight edge on part of the hair and a shaved area where something, probably a dull knife, had cut through it, leaving a tag (FIGURE 8). Within a brief period, we concluded that someone was playing games. "I'll clean up these images and then get a grad student to pull some hairs from a horse's tail at the vet school," she said. "I think there is a very good chance that these are horse hairs." Cindy called me back later that day and said that the hairs did indeed look like horse hairs (FIGURE 9).

I contacted the worried detective with the news. He had some news of his own. The town librarian had called him with a revelation. It seems that another bigfoot had surfaced some twenty-five years earlier, she recalled, and someone had written a newspaper article about it. She skimmed the local paper's archives, and lo and behold, it was the father of our new bigfoot hunter who had seen the creature's footprints a quarter of a century before. The detective went to the hunter's house and found a "foot on a stick." The hoax was revealed. Obviously, those local folks who had heard about the original bigfoot sighting had moved on or moved up. The town could return to normal—as normal as it gets in Louisiana.

With the bigfoot case down on the ledger as weirdest case of the year, I was somewhat surprised by a visit paid to me a short while later. One day, a well-dressed man stopped by my lab and asked if he could show me something he was carrying in his satchel. Reluctantly, I agreed. He explained that he had acquired the contents of the satchel from a reputable source and that he and others needed assistance in authenticating that the species was alien in nature. He had my attention.

When he opened the satchel, which smelled heavily of formalin, I saw what I believed to be two stingrays—those sea creatures that glide through the ocean waters as though they are dancing to Tchaikovsky's *Nutcracker*. The two were quite diminutive, one somewhat smaller than the other. My visitor wanted to know what I thought about them. Could they be male and female aliens? I looked at my graduate students and my look told them not to say a word. In vain, I tried to explain to the gentleman that I thought what he had were two fish. He insisted that they were aliens and that other scientists had agreed with him. I asked him where he had acquired them, and he said in a land-locked southwestern state. I immediately thought of some swampland I could sell him. He left that day, somewhat disappointed, I am sure. After his departure, I asked one of my artistic students to quickly draw what she had seen, since he had not allowed us to take photographs. The rest of us in the room agreed

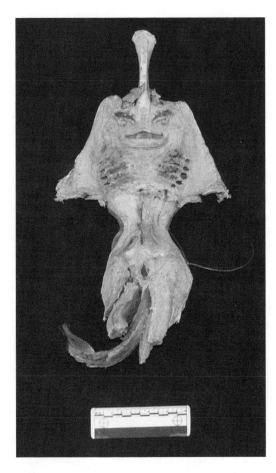

FIGURE 10.
Guitar fish

with her rendition, and all agreed that the little animals really looked like stingrays.

I went about my business for the next week or so without giving the event any consideration. But then one day the young man who helped with my yard work appeared in my driveway in his truck, and attached to the hood was a desiccated version of the little animals that had visited my lab (FIGURE 10). "For heavens sake," I thought. "Maybe they are aliens. They're everywhere."

I asked John where he had gotten his unusual hood ornament, and he replied, "From my brother. He picked it up on the beach one day and gave it to me. I just tied it to the hood of my truck for kicks. I think it's a stingray."

"Could I have it?" I asked. I told him the story and explained that the example would be great to represent unusual sightings.

"Sure," he said. "I'm tired of it anyway." He snipped the fishing line that held it to the hood of the truck and handed it over.

A few days later, LSU paleontologist Dr. Ray Wilhite came by to visit and said, "Oh, Mary, where did you get the guitar fish?" Mystery solved.

On a hot summer day in 2000, a detective from Tangipahoa Parish in the eastern part of Louisiana called with a request. A hunter walking in the woods had come across a bag with a skull and helmet. Could we look at the skull and give the sheriff's office some advice? They had an idea about it, but they wanted to confirm their thoughts. The helmet was what caught my attention. I thought, "Football? Motorcycle?" I was definitely not prepared for what was presented to me within the next hour. It was a helmet all right, but not like any I had seen in my entire career. Its origin was military, and it was old (FIGURES 11 and 12). The skull was Mongoloid, most likely Asian (FIGURE 13). They had both been found near a white plastic garbage bag deep in Louisiana's woods.

I asked one of my graduate assistants, Casey Shamblin, to get on the Web and see what he could find out about any helmet that looked like the one with which we were dealing. Within a short time, he had found one just like it. It was not a U.S.-issued helmet. In fact, it was most likely Japanese in origin, and there was a good chance that it dated to World War II.

I suggested to the sheriff's detectives that someone had apparently brought home a trophy skull from the war and, perhaps feeling a little guilty over the years and not knowing the legal ramifications of such a deed, decided he had better get rid of it. He probably just took it to a deep part of the woods and discarded it. The mystery would have been even greater if he had not discarded it in the plastic bag, as it appeared he had. Petroleum products such as the bag in question are a fairly recent phenomenon, showing up in supermarkets in abundance in the 1970s.

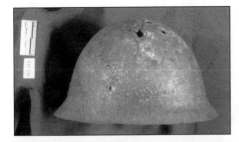

FIGURE II.
Helmet found with skull,
side view

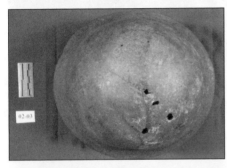

FIGURE I2.
Helmet found with skull,
top view

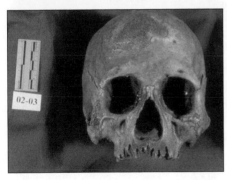

FIGURE I3.
Skull found with helmet

The sheriff decided that the age of the helmet and our analysis of the skull suggested that the time frame was outside the fifty-year range for forensic cases. They closed the case.

Unusual cases sometimes turn up in the most mundane settings. One morning, a man was walking down a street in a small community in south Louisiana when he spotted what he thought was a human skull in a ditch by the side of the road. He called the sheriff's office and they con-

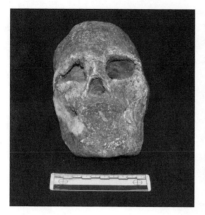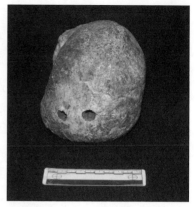

FIGURE 14.
Papier-mâché skull, front view

FIGURE 15.
Papier-mâché skull, posterior view

tacted me. I met them at the scene in less than an hour and walked to-ward the ditch in question. It was a small drainage ditch that ran parallel with the street, which was lined with houses.

A sheriff's detective pointed out the "skull" to me, and I climbed down into the three-foot-deep ditch to get a closer look. Though it looked humanlike from above, it clearly was not human. In fact, it was not even real bone. I used the tip of my trowel to touch it, and it flaked off in layers, just as I thought it would. It was papier-mâché, and a pretty good job (FIGURE 14). I cleaned the mud from it and saw that it had two holes in the back similar to holes that a bullet might make (FIGURE 15). I realized that someone must have been playing a trick on someone. However, it looked as though it had been there for a considerable period of time. The detective agreed to give it to me for my display case. He was so relieved that it wasn't real that he would have given me most anything.

Of course, the media had arrived by then and went away with just a human interest story. A few days later a former resident of the nearby street called and said she thought the skull was her son's eighth-grade art project, which she had thrown away years ago. As people do in that area, she had set her garbage can out by the street. Animals may have rooted through it, turned it over, and knocked the papier-mâché skull into the ditch. The ditch may have had mud and water in it at the time. The skull probably just settled to the bottom of the mud to be discovered years later, still intact, preserved, ironically, through a process very similar to that through which real bone might be preserved as a fossil. Rapid burial is one of the most important requisites for fossilization to occur. Otherwise, a specimen will most likely be destroyed by the taphonomic processes of scavenging and weathering.

I told the woman I hoped her son had made an A on his project. She seemed to recall that he had.

8

Tattoos and Other Body Alterations

I N 1990 in the front parking lot of a small truck stop in the city of Hammond in southeast Louisiana, the driver who was returning to his truck from his evening meal lost it soon thereafter. Lying in the parking lot was the partial body of a man. His face and much of his viscera were gone. One leg was intact, the other broken at mid shaft. The lower section of the broken leg was still inside a pair of jeans. The body was transported to the morgue. The biological profile provided by the sheriff's office noted that it was the body of a middle-aged white male. Following autopsy, the remains were taken to a small funeral home, where they were placed out back in a body bag in a shed. After the remains had lain there a few days, we were asked to assist with identifying them.

Two of my graduate students and I traveled to the funeral home to preview the body. Somewhat surprised that we were directed to an out-building behind the mortuary, we were not prepared for what we encountered when we opened the body bag that was lying on the floor of the shed. The body had been covered with lime to reduce the odor of decay. Not that unusual, but it did not stop the fly activity, which was fierce.

One of my students quickly completed drawings of nautical tattoos that were present all across the body while my other student and I worked to extract a femur and hipbones for height and for a closer age determination. From the looks of things, the skull would be of no help in getting the man identified. The entire face and a major part of the skull were missing. Officers believed the victim may have tried to hitch a ride in the wheel bed on the underbelly of an eighteen-wheeler. His left thigh terminated at mid shaft, and the end of it was smooth, as though a knife had simply sliced it in two. Ironically, the rest of that leg was still in the jeans and the foot was attached. A closer look revealed that the mid shaft of the femur was simply worn down, most likely from being dragged under the truck. His other leg was completely intact, probably caught in the wheel bed until the vehicle parked at the truck stop.

Our age evaluation back in the laboratory suggested that this white male was forty-five to fifty-five years old at the time of his death. He was approximately five feet ten inches tall and had weighed about 150–165 pounds. He was probably down on his luck at the time. He was dressed in jeans and a T-shirt and had used some type of cord as a belt to hold up his pants.

Though it has been over fourteen years since he was found in the truck stop, we believe this white male still has a chance to be identified because of his unusual tattoos and the tools now available through the Internet. The drawings reveal that he chose a nautical theme for his body art, and a few samples are shown here. One is of a female face (almost six inches long), which was on his back (FIGURE 16). She has the appearance of one of the sirens who called to the men in the mythological wanderings of heroes in ancient Greek and other writings. She might also represent an image from a ship's mast.

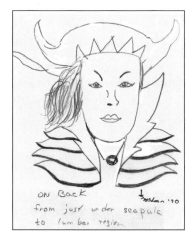

FIGURE 16.
Tattoo on man's back

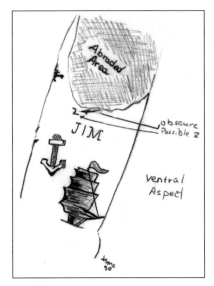

FIGURE 17.
"Jim," ship, and anchor tattoos

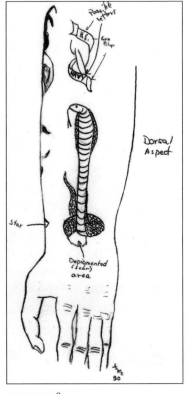

FIGURE 18.
"H. S." (or "H. M. S.") and snake
tattoos

On one arm, he had the name "Jim" (FIGURE 17) and continued the
nautical theme with a ship tattoo. The other had a snake and initials,
which might be "HS" or "HMS" (FIGURE 18). If the initials are HMS,
they may stand for Her Majesty's Ship. Could this unidentified male be a
sailor from Great Britain or Canada?

Finally, he had a mermaid on the inside of one of his calves and another female figure on the other. The second female figure looked as
though she was dressed for the cold, but with boots, a short skirt, and a
muff to warm her hands. She may represent a calendar girl from a cold
environment.

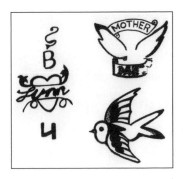

FIGURE 19.
"B 4 Lynn" and "Mother" tattoos

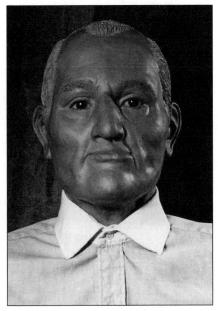

FIGURE 20.
Facial reconstruction of tattooed man

In an effort to identify the victim when he was first discovered, authorities contacted the U.S. Navy and other American military groups,
including the merchant marine, to see if they could be of help. No positive identification was ever made. His biological profile, personal history,
and DNA sample have been placed in our new Identification Data Analysis (IDA) database. Perhaps someone will help us send him home.

In April 1994, in St. James Parish in southeastern Louisiana, a nude male
body was discovered in a lightly wooded area. The man had been dead
for one to two weeks when he was found. To this day, he remains
unidentified, but, again, tattoos may hold the clue to his identity. On his
chest over each nipple is a tattoo that looks like a bluebird. His arm has
one tattoo of a broken heart, with "B 4 Lynn" incorporated into the design, and another that reads "Mother" (FIGURE 19).

The victim also had a wire in his left knee that suggests he had undergone reconstructive surgery, perhaps to repair torn ligaments. Finally, Eileen Barrow completed a facial reconstruction of the man (FIGURE 20). The reconstruction was publicized locally, but no one came forward with a name. The identifying traits of this man, too, will be listed in the IDA database.

Though these two cases represent extremes in which multiple body tattoos have not resulted in a positive identification, other cases have been solved through the use of tattoos. Tattoos of women's names, the person's nickname, and everything from Woody Woodpecker to teardrops cascading down the person's cheek have all been helpful in identifying victims. With the popularity of tattooing these days, in part as a result of the relaxation of the stigma attached to it in the past, at the FACES Lab we always keep in mind that if any skin is still present on the body, we will use bleach diluted with water to look for those hidden identifiers. We have learned that tattoos can be present absolutely anywhere on the body where there is skin. Nothing surprises us in this regard.

Tattoos are just one example of physical evidence associated with a body that can lead to a positive identification. In one case on which we worked, the body of an elderly woman was found near her car in an isolated, wooded region just off an old logging road close to a main highway. Authorities felt that she may have become disoriented and taken a wrong turn, driving her car deeper and deeper into the woods. She may have died from shock or exposure, exacerbated by her advanced age and frail health. They knew who she was, they said, based on the car and personal belongings found near her body, but, legally, they had to have a positive identification. Detectives found out from family members that she had recently undergone knee surgery. They brought her body to our lab, and we excised the metal prosthesis that had been placed in her knee. Since the surgery was fairly recent, identifying numbers on the metal plate were directly traced to her and offered strong evidence of positive identification. Her family could bury her with utmost confidence that she was their loved one.

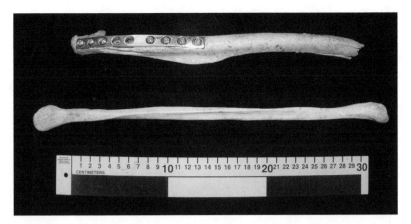

FIGURE 21.
Animal bone with rods *(top)* and human fibula

As an added twist to the identification puzzle, occasionally, prosthetic devices are also found in animals that become our cases when the authorities are presented with isolated bones. Many people are surprised at the expense others will go to in order to save a prized pet. Usually, animals with prosthetics have come to be seen as members of the family—but not always!

A few years ago, officers arrived at my laboratory with a fairly substantial bone that had a large metal rod in it. Clearly it was not human, but the human bone it most closely resembled was a fibula, the thin outer bone in the lower leg (FIGURE 21). To make identification of the species even more difficult, remodeling of the bone around the metal rod distorted the bone's normal shape. I decided this was a mystery for our friend, paleontologist Dr. Ray Wilhite. Dr. Wilhite studied it for a while and determined that it was the wing, or humerus, of an ostrich. Now what in the world was an ostrich humerus doing in a lightly wooded pasture in south Louisiana? In fact this mystery was easily explained, and not with the "only in Louisiana" theorem, tempting as it was.

We did a little checking on our "victim" and discovered that in the 1980s ostrich meat was being touted across the country as the "new white meat." Naturally, Louisiana's subtropical climate was an ideal setting for an ostrich farm, where everyone was going to get rich quick. Ostriches are not cheap, costing many thousands of dollars. We decided that one of the costly ostriches had broken his wing, either accidentally or in a fight with another ostrich or, perhaps, with Louisiana's fictional wolf-man, the *loup-garou*, whose presence is legend in Louisiana's folklore. Regardless of how he broke the wing, the ostrich represented a sizeable investment, and his wing had to be repaired.

Eventually (actually fairly quickly) the new white meat went the way of many strangely unpopular ventures—straight out the window. The animal then either died of natural causes or perhaps, unfortunately, was eaten by his master. Even the feral dogs and pigs in the area could not eat the metal rod. Similar prosthetic devices have made their way to our lab attached to the long bones of other animals, especially large dogs, but, I admit, the ostrich case is my favorite.

Tattoos and prosthetic devices provide valuable assistance in identifying humans and sometimes even their pets. Though our main job is to examine human bones and aid law enforcement agencies with positive identifications, we often receive skeletal remains with no prosthetic devices which have to be identified as human or nonhuman. The advent of e-mail and digital photography has helped tremendously in this effort and has saved an unimaginable amount of time for both law enforcement officers and us. The bones that are provided for such analysis usually have been found in an area where an individual disappeared or where foul play was suspected. We receive approximately ten or more such cases each year. Determining whether a set of remains is human or nonhuman plays a strategic role in any missing person case in which search efforts are directed to a particular geographic location.

The following photographs of human and nonhuman bones help illustrate how forensic anthropologists answer one of the most important questions they address: "Are these human bones?"

FIGURE 22 compares a human clavicle, the collar bone, to a bone that is often misidentified as human, an alligator femur. Remarkably, the alligator femur, or thighbone, looks a lot like a human collar bone. It is somewhat larger than a typical clavicle, but we have seen some human clavicles that rival this particular example in size.

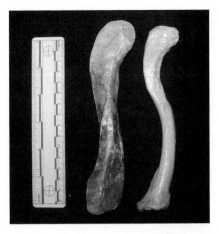

FIGURE 22.
Human clavicle *(right)* and
alligator femur

FIGURE 23 is a photograph comparing some of the bones of the forepaw of a bear with the corresponding bones in a human hand. The bear's bones are similar in appearance to the human's, and one can see how easily the bear's forepaw could be mistaken for part of a human hand, especially if tissue were still present, as it was in the case illustrated here. The partial paw was found in a wooded area in north Louisiana and had been chewed on by wild animals. Law enforcement agents correctly called us and asked for our assistance in determining if the remains were human or not. First we x-rayed the remains, and then we removed the putrefactive tissue.

Generally speaking, the carpals, the first group of bones in the hand, have a different shape in humans than those of the bear, and the bear's carpals are smaller. Also, the metacarpals in a human hand—those short, tubular bones just beyond the carpals—exhibit more variation in the thickness and shape of the shaft than do the bear's. The distal ends of the bear's metacarpals (the portions of each of those tubular bones of the forepaw farthest from the wrist) also have a different shape from the distal ends of the human metacarpals.

Finally, FIGURE 24 is a photograph of the upper dental arcades of a human and a pig. Pigs' teeth are shaped more like humans than are those of most animals one typically encounters in forensics work. Since feral pigs are present in the woods of Louisiana and many other states, teeth

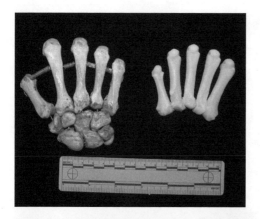

FIGURE 23.
Partial bear's forepaw *(right)*
and human finger bones

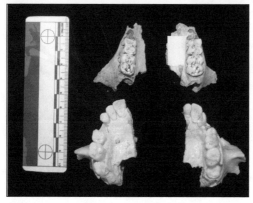

FIGURE 24.
Upper teeth of pig *(top)*
and human

assumed to be those of pigs need to be examined by forensic anthropologists to make sure they are not human.

9

Precious Doe

FBI Agent Sue Stiltner arrived at my office one day in 2002. She was in Baton Rouge to consult on an FBI case and asked David Smith, a detective with the East Baton Rouge Parish sheriff's office, if he knew me. He told her that he did and that he would arrange for her to meet me. When she got to the FACES Lab, she told me she had heard a lot about our lab and the work that we do. She was especially interested in our research on three-dimensional facial reconstruction and our studies on tissue depth thicknesses in living persons. I explained that research project to her, how we had gathered considerable tissue depth data using noninvasive ultrasound on both sexes, various races, and a wide range of ages. Sue wanted to hear more about our work with children, and I told her that we had scanned more than eight hundred volunteers ranging in age from three to ninety-seven.

"So, where is this going, Sue?" I asked her, knowing full well that she would not be wasting her valuable time just chitchatting in my lab, as interesting as I thought it might be.

"Mary," she said, "Kansas City, Missouri, is one of the regions in my jurisdiction. Have you heard of the Precious Doe case up there?" Actually, I had. It was a case that had stayed in the national headlines for several days back in the spring of 2002. I remembered it, but I asked her to refresh my memory.

A sheriff's deputy was walking along a small dirt road in a wooded region in the heart of Kansas City, Missouri. He was looking for a missing man. He noticed an area very near the edge of the road where flies were circling all about. He knew immediately that something was dead. What he was not prepared for was the sight of a small child's body, definitely female, lying near the edge of the road. She had no head. He immediately called the police. Crime scene personnel reached the scene in record time. The detectives and volunteers continued looking in the general area, hoping to find the child's head. They were not successful. The next day, an older black male announced to passersby that he was going into the woods to look for the head. No one would have dreamed that he could find it. A television reporter just happened to be in the immediate area doing a follow-up story on the little girl and captured the man picking up a plastic bag that was alive with flies. It seemed a strange coincidence that the man just happened to want to look for the little girl's head and then found it so easily. After checking out his background, law enforcement personnel eliminated him as a suspect, but the city was in an uproar. Everyone was upset because no one could identify the child. How could they solve the case if they did not know who she was?

The entire community came forward to try to help identify the child. Somewhere along the way, they began to call the small victim "Precious Doe" rather than Jane Doe, the moniker typically assigned to unidentified females. "Precious Doe" made the case seem more personal and seemed more fitting for a child.

The autopsy performed by the chief medical examiner in Missouri confirmed that the body was that of a black female, exact age unknown, but most likely between three and seven years old. The autopsy report also noted that she had been dead for only a day or so when found. However, because of the rapid decay of her soft tissue in the heat, due in part to her size, her face was unrecognizable.

A two-dimensional line drawing was completed and publicized nationwide. Then another. No results. Next, authorities decided to try a three-dimensional facial reconstruction. They sent the skull to a forensic sculptor in Pennsylvania and publicized the results. No luck again. Hundreds of phone calls had not provided any real leads. Who was this child? Didn't anyone know her? Did someone have a little girl and then suddenly not have her anymore? Did the mother or father claim she was "visiting relatives" in a distant state?

The poignant case history was what troubled Agent Sue Stiltner. Over a period of months, Agent Stiltner became friends with Sgt. David Bernard, a lifelong resident of the Kansas City area and the senior detective on the case. Dave had more than twenty-five years' experience in law enforcement and had collected two large file cabinet drawers of evidence, leads, speculation, and anything else he could get his hands on that might be remotely linked to Precious Doe. He personally had fielded hundreds of calls on the tip line and checked out all those with any potential.

The citizens of Kansas City donated a casket in which Precious Doe could be buried. A funeral home waived all fees, and someone else donated a plot in a local cemetery. Near the scene where her body had been found, mourners erected a shrine in her honor. They filled the area protected by a canvas tent with toys, mementos, and posters of the various artists' sketches of Precious Doe. They went there daily for candlelight memorials. Finally, they buried her in the white casket in the donated cemetery plot. On her tombstone, they carved the name "Precious Doe."

But Sue Stiltner could not let the case rest. Not only had such a vile act been committed against an innocent child, but that child still did not have a real name. I never dreamed that the FACES Lab would have the opportunity to help on the case. Before Sue could ask the question I knew she was going to ask, I threw my double punch. "Sue," I asked, "do you think there's a chance we could exhume the body and try one more facial reconstruction?" She knew she had me then. Of course, she had me when she first mentioned Precious Doe, but I didn't want to always seem so eager. I, too, had thought about Precious Doe over the months following her discovery. I had reviewed the images of her on the Web and had asked our forensic sculptor, Eileen Barrow, what she thought of them. Never one to criticize the work of others, Eileen spoke more about the age of one of them, noting that the image looked a little too mature for such a young child. We also agreed that the clothing on the mature image seemed out of place on the little girl. Though her exact age was unknown, three to seven years was fairly broad as an age estimation.

Children are aged through dental development, which is apparent from x-rays. Often, you can get a very tight age range by looking at the growth stage of their deciduous teeth, or baby teeth, and any permanent teeth that may have begun to develop.

Sue, Eileen, and I had a long discussion about Precious Doe. Sue gave me Sergeant Bernard's telephone number and e-mail address, and Dave and I began a correspondence that would continue for more than six months before he was able to secure permission to exhume Precious Doe's body. During that time, I thought about how we could help in the case.

Precious Doe's age was problematic in her identification. If she were at least five, she would probably be in some school system's records. Someone might have noted if a child were unaccounted for. But if she were younger than that, as I had thought from the beginning, she might have slipped through the cracks without any public agency knowing anything about her. We hoped for the former but felt it might be the latter.

The medical examiner's office in Kansas City had already secured a sample of Precious Doe's DNA, and the FBI had analyzed it and entered the results into its database. In fact her DNA had been compared to the family members of a child missing from Florida, Rilya Wilson. Authorities hoped they could clear up two cases, but instead neither was solved. Precious Doe remained unidentified, and Rilya Wilson was still missing.

On the one-year anniversary of Precious Doe's discovery, national attention once again focused on her. Still no leads. Dave Bernard had been working behind the scenes to get permission to exhume her body. Additionally, a national television production company wanted to do a special program on her if we actually exhumed her body. In June 2003, Dave called me with the exciting news. Everything had been taken care of. Could I come the next week? I made reservations immediately.

The plan was that I would fly to Kansas City, be present to supervise the exhumation, and return to Louisiana with Precious Doe's skull. We would reexamine her skull at the FACES Lab, and I would also take it to the LSU dental school in New Orleans for Dr. Robert Barsley and his colleagues to x-ray her teeth with their digital x-ray machine, the new buzz at the time in dentistry. Digital x-rays can capture all of the subtle bumps, curves, fissures, and other anomalies that individualize a person's dental morphology with amazing precision, so we had good reason to hope for a more precise determination of Precious Doe's age.

Dave met me at the airport in Kansas City. I was standing in line waiting to get my baggage, and I saw this rather serious looking man with blond hair pacing back and forth in the waiting area. We caught each other's eyes and nodded at one another. I knew that he was Sgt. David Bernard. Early the next morning he picked me up at the hotel, and we quickly traveled to the cemetery. Local and national news media were everywhere. Dave had arranged for them to be stationed a considerable distance from the actual exhumation. I had participated in several exhumations and knew that raising a casket could take a fairly long time and also could reveal some things, such as water leakage, that should not be captured on film.

The cemetery crew skillfully raised the adult-sized white metal casket from the burial pit and loaded it onto the truck for the trip to the medical examiner's office. I was somewhat surprised at such a large casket for such a small child but remembered that it had been donated. Following the exhumation, Dave and I participated in a news conference. I had already anticipated the anxious reporters' questions. "What do you plan to do that has not already been done before?" one of them asked immediately.

I focused on the fact that we all needed to see if we could pinpoint Precious Doe's age a little more closely, explaining the importance of estimating her age as accurately and precisely as possible. I also told them of our research on tissue depth thicknesses in small children and our laboratory's successes with identifications from clay facial reconstructions. Emphasizing that we did not have a magic wand for identifying Precious Doe, I explained that Dave, Sue, and I wanted to try everything humanly possible to evaluate her remains one more time to see if we could identify her.

At the medical examiner's office, the technicians unsealed the casket and I stared at Precious Doe for the first time. As a female and a mother, I was not exactly pleased with the way she had been positioned inside the casket, but that was secondary. I gently examined her body and made notes about the specifics of her remains, notes I knew I could never share.

Early the next morning, I caught a flight back to Baton Rouge with her skull resting in a case beside me. Airport authorities in Kansas City had been very cooperative when Dave had asked for a special private security screening of Precious Doe's skull so that it did not have to be subjected to the usual public x-ray machine.

The next week, I traveled to the LSU dental school in New Orleans and was greeted by Dr. Barsley and several senior faculty members, all anxious to assist with the dental evaluation of Precious Doe. Dr. Barsley attached her skull to the digital x-ray machine with tape, positioning it in the proper anatomical plane. Unfortunately, the machine was not designed for such a small skull or one that had no tissue on it. Living patients were the machine's usual subjects. The specialists tried over and over again to get a good image on the $25,000 machine, but no luck. We finally resorted to traditional x-rays so that all of the attending dentists could have input into Precious Doe's age estimate before we left the school. Interestingly, those age estimates varied somewhat according to which professor you asked. Dr. Barsley and I still maintained that she was most likely between two and a half and three and a half years old. One could easily see the stage of development of her deciduous molars and the beginnings of her first premolars (the teeth that would replace her baby molars). Since the enamel develops first and then the root, those stages of growth can be used to estimate chronological age. Precious Doe had her two deciduous molars in each of her four quadrants, but she also had permanent molars in their early stages of development. Though the age estimates suggested by the professors ranged from three to six, Dr. Barsley's estimate would be the one we would work with. Unlike all the other professors at the meeting that day, he had examined literally thousands of dental x-rays over the years for positive identifications. He and I felt confident that Precious Doe was between two and a half and three and a half years of age.

We are currently working with one of my graduate students to examine x-rays of hundreds of children of various ages, both sexes, and different races to determine if there have been changes in the rates of growth of teeth. Though the growth and development of teeth are considered to be more genetically controlled than the growth of the rest of the human skeleton (which can be affected greatly by lack of proper food), some researchers have suggested that the development of teeth is more plastic than once thought.

Once we returned to the FACES Lab, we conducted a careful analysis of Precious Doe's skull to look for any evidence of perimortem trauma or other anomalies that could help law enforcement in their hunt for her killer. Those results were provided to Dave and his team.

Our final task was to create an image of what she may have looked like in life. Eileen Barrow glued the twenty-one tissue depth markers across her skull. The length of those markers was based on our previous research results for black female children. Our data are the most complete that are currently available for children. Eileen then positioned the skull on a metal rod anchored to a twelve-inch wooden base. Then we called Dr. Warren Wagguesback, an expert in computer engineering. Dr. Wagguesback had been working with us to create a computer program with special coordinate capabilities that would allow us to build faces with the aid of a computer rather than clay. His graduate students came to the laboratory and scanned Precious Doe's skull and entered that scan into their database. Eventually, with the software they hoped to develop, a special "printer" would take that information and create a three-dimensional image of what the face might look like. At this stage, they could already print, or build, a model of the skull from synthetic material, but they could not add a face to it. Though others across the country are working on similar research, no one has yet developed a three-dimensional imaging program that rivals what clay can do if handled by the right artist. That is the key.

On the other hand, the software Dr. Wagguesback and his students were developing could generate a plastic model of a skull, which a forensic sculptor could use rather than the actual skull to build a face. That would protect fragile bones. Additionally, their software could fill in missing bone on a skull. For example, a skull with a missing right cheekbone could be scanned and the printer could create a mirror image of the left cheekbone that was present and direct it to the area of missing bone. This would be especially helpful in cases involving extensive trauma from high velocity, blunt force, or fire.

Widespread interest in the art of facial reconstruction will allow other

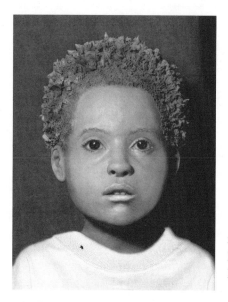

FIGURE 25.
Facial reconstruction of Precious
Doe

researchers working with MRIs and CAT scans to create a three-dimensional image of a face from just a skull at some point in the near future.
Will that image be more accurate than the three-dimensional clay facial
reconstruction? Probably not, but it certainly would be faster. Expedi-
ency can be important in some situations. Currently, we continue to use
the three-dimensional clay technique that has been successful for us in
the past.

After Dr. Wagguesback finished scanning Precious Doe's skull, Eileen
protected the nasal opening and deep eye orbits with cotton wadding.
Then she began to add clay across the face area. In a matter of a week,
Precious Doe had another face. Eileen photographed the image and
scanned that photo into Photoshop to begin making the image more life-
like. The hairline and hair style were based on morgue photos of Precious
Doe's hair, which Eileen saw only after she had finished the face. She always wants to see any images only after completing reconstructive work,
in order to avoid being biased by them. Her three-dimensional image of
Precious Doe (FIGURE 25) is somewhat different from those created by

the others, but there is still no guarantee that this one best represents what Precious Doe looked like in life.

Sgt. David Bernard came to Louisiana and hand-carried the three-dimensional image back to Kansas City for a news conference that we hoped would generate new leads. He actually purchased an extra seat on the plane for Precious Doe so that the clay image would not be damaged (even though that was highly unlikely, since he also placed the reconstruction in a sturdy wooden carrying case that was patterned after a design we developed). The new image was posted on the Kansas City Police Department's web site.

On May 4, 2005, Precious Doe was identified. After four long years she had a name: Erica Michelle Maria Green. Erica was three years old when she died. She was reburied in Kansas City, and her real name is on her grave marker. A special service was held for her. I was there.

.

10

Unidentified Homicide Victim

I T was the summer of 2001 when we watched the backhoe pull up to the grave in the corner of the small rural cemetery in Greens-burg, Louisiana. Detective Dennis Stewart with the Louisiana State Police was almost twitching with excitement, and so was I. In 1979, when the victim was first buried, I was an undergraduate at Louisiana State University with two small children. I was an English major at the time, and nothing was further from my mind than identifying or digging up bodies. Dennis, on the other hand, was just a kid in 1979 and was haunted by this case, so haunted that when he became a detective years later, he wanted to try to do something about it. On the tombstone, the epitaph read, UNIDENTIFIED HOMICIDE VICTIM.

Dennis had contacted me at the LSU FACES Laboratory a couple of years prior to the day of the exhumation to ask for my help in the case. We often get requests for assistance in opening graves, but usually nothing ever comes of the initial inquiry. Something about this young man who had dedicated his life to helping others made me think this case would be different. For years, Dennis felt as though he had been spinning his wheels, waiting for just the right permission and support to fall into place in order to exhume the body. For such an exhumation to occur, a judge had to sign the order, and there had to be "just cause" to remove a person from his or her grave. What bothered Dennis about this case was something that bothered me—something, in fact, that nags at me constantly when I get a case until it is resolved. One of the most important things I can do as a forensic anthropologist is to identify a victim so that the family can go on with their lives. The teenager whose remains now rested several feet below the surface in the metal transport box doubling as a casket had not been allowed that small dignity. He was unidentified. Dennis and I knew it, the locals knew it, and now the judge knew it. He agreed to allow the exhumation. It would be worth it to try to give this child a name. In 1979 some of the tools and technology for identifying the teenager were not available. One of my greatest worries was that the incredible tools of the twenty-first century still might not be enough.

I did not know what to expect as the recovery team reached the small, donated metal burial box in which the teenager had been laid to rest. Anything that I might do to help Dennis was predicated on good preservation of remains. In the subtropical climate of south Louisiana, I knew we were asking a lot.

The workers were prison trustees on work release. Though they said nothing at all as they worked (probably because they had been told to), I saw questions in their eyes. A television crew captured the exhumation for the evening news, but after more than twenty-five years since the original discovery of the child's body, publicity might only result in a mild curiosity from the television viewing audience.

As part of a cold case review, this teenage John Doe had been publicized on flyers in recent years. A morgue photo (FIGURE 26) had been enhanced at the National Center for Missing and Exploited Children (NCMEC) and was posted on the Louisiana State Police Web site with the following message:

> Request for Assistance!
> Unknown Homicide Victim
> Age: 15–19
> Found: 11-12-79
> Race: White
> Sex: Male
> Hair: Blond
> Eyes: Blue or Gray
> Height: 5′5″
> Weight: 125 lbs.

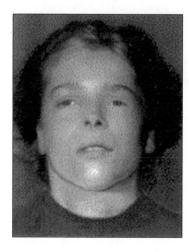

FIGURE 26.
"Unidentified Homicide Victim"

Victim was found in St. Helena Parish near Greensburg, Louisiana. Physical markings on the victim included: X or + sign on the left hand between the thumb and index finger; a vertical surgical scar at the top of the navel measuring three inches; and a prominent scar on the right hand beginning on the knuckle of the middle finger and ending on the knuckle of the little finger which measures 2.5 inches. The victim's blood type is O.

What could we possibly hope to add to this very thorough and incredibly detailed description? For one thing, Dennis had recently received a serious inquiry from a woman in the northeastern United States who thought that the child might be her son. DNA identification was only a dream back in 1979. Also, no dental chart was prepared for the victim at that time. At the very least, a DNA sample, if possible, and a dental chart could be two important tools for possible identification. If he were not exhumed, he would never be identified. By exhuming his body, we hoped we could get that DNA sample to compare to one from the anxious mother. Additionally, we could compare the DNA profile and dental x-rays to those of other missing teenagers if the mother's sample was not a match. There was some discussion of a clay facial reconstruction, but I could not imagine that any image we could provide would be better than the morgue photo that had been enhanced by NCMEC. Besides, the condition of the remains after so long might make this a moot point.

As the crew finished uncovering the donated metal transport box, my worst fears were realized: holes had rusted through the box, and water poured from it when the crew raised it from the burial pit. Dennis looked at me with disappointed eyes. I smiled a weakly optimistic smile at the bleak evidence and motioned for the crew to continue raising the box. Until we knew the extent of damage to the contents, I would not believe that all was lost.

The trustees loaded the fragile metal box into the back of our vehicle, and Dennis and I agreed to open it the next day. If remains were still present, the sooner we could get them out of the damaged box the better, as exposure to the air could accelerate deterioration. Though I did not tell Dennis, the lack of odor emanating from the box did not bode well for preservation, but I would wait until the next day to see.

Dennis was at our lab early the next morning. A good night's sleep had put a positive spin on his enthusiasm as well as mine. After several minutes of frustrating hammering to dislodge the stubborn screws, we finally had to cut them away. As we raised the lid, my heart sank. The metal box was filled with mud. Bones protruded from the mud here and there, their integrity greatly compromised. But where was the skull? Near one end, I saw bits and pieces of it sticking out of the mud. I knew any formal reconstruction was not possible. I also knew what Dennis's first question would be: "Mary, will we be able to find any intact DNA?"

"I don't know, Dennis, but we will darn sure try," was the best I could do. I explained to him that it would take a week or so to clean up the bones and evaluate the remains. I suggested that he retreat and allow us to do our job and said that we would call him back soon. I understood his concern. He had waited all of his life for this. I told him that the minute we finished our evaluation, he would be the first to know.

Slowly, we removed the fragile bones from the mud. They were extremely soft because the water, having most likely filled the box on many occasions since the metal rusted away, had accelerated the destruction of the bone. The leaching process had made it soft and limber, almost like rubber. Minimally, we had to let it dry out under the fume hood to try to preserve it as well as possible. All the long bones had fragmented ends. The ends of those bones are composed of what we refer to as "trabecular" or "spongy" bone, which is more porous than the denser, more compact bone of the shafts.

On one count, however, I was very pleased. The teeth were intact, and many were still present in their sockets. Not only could we do a dental chart, some teeth might also contain DNA. The bone surrounding them may have protected them over the years. For the first time in several days, I had hope. Added to that encouraging note was the presence of multiple fillings in his jaw. This young teenager had experienced good dental care as a child. Someone, probably his mother, had made certain of that.

For two days, we allowed the bones to dry under the fume hood. As they dried, their outer, cortical layer began to separate from the rest of the bone. Their appearance was very similar to that of historic remains I had recovered from moist environments in Louisiana. If long-term preservation of the entire skeleton had been our goal, we would have used hypodermic needles filled with a preservative known as "gelva" to impregnate the bone. This "gelva" is a mixture of polyvinyl acetate beads and ethyl alcohol. However, this was a forensic case in which identifying the victim was our goal, not a historic research project.

Our subsequent dental chart and x-rays revealed that the teenager indeed had several fillings. The development of his third molars, his wisdom teeth, suggested an age between fourteen and sixteen. Somewhere there might be dental records and x-rays on this child.

Within days, we had generated our profile, which basically agreed with that of the pathologist from a quarter of a century earlier. Young white male, fourteen to sixteen years of age. We sampled his remains for DNA, and a few weeks later, the lab results confirmed that DNA could be extracted from the material and that a profile was possible. Dennis obtained a DNA sample from the mother with the missing son. Unfortunately, Dennis had to call the mother shortly thereafter with the disappointing news: the young teenager was not her son. Though this finding was initially frustrating, this teenage victim now has a chance to be identified that he did not have before. If we had not exhumed his body, he would have remained unidentified in perpetuity. Now he waits in my lab for someone to take him home. I hope someday someone will.

Mardi Gras Man

OFFICER Mula's voice on the other end of the phone resonated with the rich French ancestry of so many of the law enforcement agents with whom I had worked over the last twenty-plus years in south Louisiana. He was calling about a case in St. Mary Parish that had frustrated all of us for more than two years. The victim was a white male between thirty-five and forty-five years of age whose body had been discovered when parish road crews were dredging ditches along the highway to prevent flooding.

"Mary, I may have a lead on Mardi Gras Man. Could you pull your file on him?" The victim had been dubbed "Mardi Gras Man" by the news media because we had found a string of cheap yellow Mardi Gras beads with his remains. Mardi Gras in Louisiana, usually celebrated in February each year, is one of the biggest parties in the world and is punctuated by the distribution of millions of cheap plastic beads thrown from floats by often drunken riders and caught by sometimes less-than-sober parade-goers. A month prior to Mardi Gras, the Mardi Gras beads begin to show up at various parties and parades. Gooey king cakes, each containing a one-inch tall, naked plastic baby, and adding inches to midriffs already thickened by the Christmas holidays, are sold by the thousands (if you get the baby, you buy the cake the next week). Meanwhile, many locals finalize plans to leave the area. A week or so after Mardi Gras is over, signaled by Fat Tuesday and the beginning of Lent, the beads go underground again. Though some may be seen dangling from the rearview mirrors of automobiles for weeks to come, most people put theirs away until the next year.

The day we had retrieved Case 00-25, Mardi Gras had not been on my mind. It was a late-September morning in 2000 when I got a call from Bob Bizet, Dr. Chip Metz's chief coroner's investigator. "We need your help, Mary. Can you come? I'll tell you all about it when you get here."

"Of course we can come," I told Bob. "Give us a couple of hours and we'll be there." The ride to St. Mary Parish would take at least an hour and a half. That meant I had thirty minutes before I had to walk out the door. I hurried down the hall to the office of my research associate, Beth Basset. Beth gathered together the crew of graduate students we assemble for each case. Our labor force always depends on who's available and how much time each student needs to mobilize. The numbers increase or decrease according to the location of the case, scheduling conflicts with the students' classes, and the condition of the remains. On such a cold, rainy day, our numbers would not be large.

We mustered three enthusiastic graduate students eager to gain the experience so coveted in this field and took off down the highway with various tools and equipment bulging from the back of our new Suburban dubbed "Belle." Belle had been purchased with monies allocated by the state legislature to replace "Blue," a worthy vehicle that had been donated by the local sheriff's office when it reached 200,000 miles and was currently in sickbay. We always name our vehicles and accept the gentle ribbing when officers find out that "Belle" is actually our suburban rather than one of our graduate students.

As we neared the scene, its location was obvious. We were approximately five miles east of Morgan City along Highway 182. More than fifteen vehicles with lights spinning stretched along the highway and adjacent to a service road that ran parallel to the highway. Small groups of detectives and uniformed officers parted like waves to let us through. Many smiled and waved, their faces looking all too familiar. They pointed the way to the victim, and one look confirmed their discovery: bones and clothing protruded from the large pile of wet mud and debris hanging from the jaws of the backhoe.

We had already given the victim a number, 00-25, our twenty-fifth case to date in the year 2000. Our first task would be to recover as many of the remains as possible and then provide our usual profile of age, sex, race, height, and postmortem interval, or time since death. It had been raining continuously for hours. Though it slowed to a drizzle, we would all be covered in mud before the day was over.

Bob gave me a quick rundown on what they had found and how they had discovered the remains. The backhoe operator had been dredging the ditch up and down the highway in an effort to ease drainage problems in the area. As he maneuvered the bucket toward a fallen log to get it out of the way, he hit the body. He did not realize what he had in his bucket until he swung it around to dump the load on the growing mound of dirt along the highway. As the slush began to fall from the bucket, he saw the bones and what looked like clothing clinging to the lip of the bucket. He stopped all forward motion, turned off his engine, and called headquarters.

When we inspected the backhoe, some of the human remains were still hanging from the bucket. Other bones were resting in a pile on top of the mud mound. One look and I knew that Belle would need a thorough bath when we got home. So would I. I climbed onto the pile of wet mud and debris and picked up a hipbone. It was basically clean, and I recognized the sex immediately—narrow sciatic notch, acute subpubic angle, no ventral arc, broad medial-lateral border in the subpubic region, small pelvic inlet: male, no doubt.

Though the surface on the auricular region of the hip would need cleaning before analysis, the symphyseal face of the pubic bone was mud free. The ridges and undulations associated with youth were gone, with only a vestige of billowing. The symphyseal face exhibited a rim around its margins. The man was definitely over thirty-five. Fairly quickly, we knew the answers to two of the three most important questions: sex, age, and race. An accurate assessment of race would require the skull. "Where is the skull?" I asked.

"We have not seen one yet," they told me. That was not what I wanted to hear, but I would deal with it later. I put a couple of students to work on the debris pile. The remains were so disturbed by the backhoe bucket that mapping of that group of bones would consist of draw-ing a circle to represent the jumbled bones and clothing that were present in the backhoe debris. We would link that group of bones to any others we found that were not disturbed.

Beth and I then began to evaluate what we thought to be the original location of the remains. The body had at one time rested immediately adjacent to a log crossing the ditch, the same log the backhoe operator had attempted to remove. When he lowered his bucket to pick up the log, he grabbed the body first. Partial remains lay in a pile under the log, but no skull.

We searched in the immediate area adjacent to the woods, but the mosquitoes were fierce that day. It had stopped raining by then and what seemed like hundreds of them came at us as we ventured into the woods. We decided to wait a while to see if they would subside. We worked for several hours to map and recover all the obvious skeletal remains we could find. However, just as we completed the mapping, the rain re-turned in torrents, and it was getting dark. I told the investigators that there was a chance that an animal had dragged the skull into the woods. I felt the best thing we could do was to return the next day to look for the skull; hopefully, the rain would have subsided by then. The next morn-ing, a phone call from Bob Bizet solved the immediate problem.

"We found the skull, Mary," he said, "just inside the woods, but not the lower jaw. I'm bringing it to you now."

Needless to say, we were glad we did not have to go back into the woods. By the time Bob arrived, we had cleaned the mud from the bones and laid out the recovered remains in anatomical order. Two-thirds of the skeleton was present. Some of the lower arm and hand bones were miss-ing, which was not at all surprising. Two things could have happened. Those dangling parts could have been lost in the ditch, especially if the body had been transported for a way down the ditch. We had no idea where the body actually originated in the area. Rains and flooding could have driven it down the ditch for hundreds if not thousands of feet, and obviously something (or someone) had carried away the skull—some-thing big, I assumed, since it made the effort to take the skull, an element that is hard to hold, when other, smaller bones lay nearby. It may also have carried away the other missing parts of the skeleton. Those parts were probably lost forever. Just to know that the skull had been found was a great relief. Now we could also evaluate the race of the individual and feel comfortable with our assessment. A few formulae exist for assessing the variation between white and black individuals based on the anterior/posterior curvature of the femoral shaft and other regions in the proximal femur. However, those techniques are not nearly as accurate as the assessment of a complete skull.

Bob arrived at our lab in record time. I knew immediately that we had the remains of a white male: sloping eye orbits; a narrow, pinched nasal opening; a fairly straight midface profile when viewed in the lateral position. Measurements at strategic points across the skull were entered into FORDISC, and we printed the results, which overwhelmingly indicated a white male. As noted previously, our initial evaluation suggested he was between thirty-five and forty-five years of age, and he was between five feet six inches and five feet nine inches tall. Judging from the advanced stage of decomposition, I calculated that he had been dead for a minimum of several months, possibly more. He had only a little tissue left on his body and some adipocere, the waxy material that was the result of the hydrolysis, or separation, of body fats in a moist environment.

Often people ask, "Well, what happened to him? How did he get in that ditch?" Evidence on his body suggested that he may have been injured slightly at or near the time of death. If he were hitchhiking along the road late at night, he may have been a victim of a hit and run. Someone out there may know exactly why he was in the ditch.

Identifying him was a different story. His dental status was good in the upper jaw. With only that to go on, identifying him would be somewhat problematic. He had almost perfect teeth, with no fillings, but the last two molars on the upper right side (numbers 1 and 2) had been removed sometime before death, and the bone looked as though it might be in the process of healing, or remodeling. Since he had no fillings, which people his age typically might have, identification from dental x-rays might not be possible. However, he had probably seen a dentist in recent years to remove the two back teeth. He also had a very wide space, or diastema, between his two upper front teeth, his central incisors. A smiling photograph of a possible match would most likely show that space and could be used to identify this man. Another important, identifying fact about this young man is that he must have sustained some injuries a few weeks or months prior to his death. He had healing fractures in his thoracic vertebrae and in some of his ribs. He may have been in a fight in recent months, or, perhaps, he had fallen and sustained an injury on a job.

His clothing was something else altogether. He was dressed in a way that suggested he was experiencing rather grim economic times in his life. His Nike shoes were very worn, and the soles were tied together. He was wearing blue pants with the Levi's label inside, size 36. He had on a beige cotton jacket with plaid lining and a blue Sears vest. He had no identifying papers on his body. And, finally, he wore Mardi Gras beads around his neck. I often thought of these details in the months that followed, wondering if we would ever learn who this man was.

When Officer Mula called me that December day in 2002, he had heard from a couple from out of state that they thought the man was their son. Everything fit, they said. Their son had been down on his luck and living somewhere in the Morgan City area, they thought. Mula asked for my help in getting a DNA profile of the victim. He wished to compare it to that of the family members. I submitted a piece of one of the long bones and a tooth. Carolyn Booker, DNA specialist at the Acadiana Crime Lab in New Iberia, Louisiana, called us with the results: no match. I couldn't believe it. Just when you think you have a case solved, something happens that reduces your chances of sending a person home.

We have not given up on this case. We will identify this man and send him home, not today, perhaps, or even tomorrow, but we will do it. I have to believe that. No one should linger in a vault in my lab indefinitely. That I will not tolerate. As other leads come our way, we continue to check them out and hope for the day when we can give Mardi Gras Man a real name and send him home. Until then, he and others similar to him wait in my lab, their biological and DNA profiles part of our new IDA database.

12

Unexpected Cargo

THE railroad tank car loomed ahead of me. It looked much larger up close than such cars do when you see them rolling along the track in a long chain pulled by a powerful locomotive.

The call had come in the early afternoon. A detective had a bone he wanted me to evaluate. He was certain it was human, but he wanted my opinion to confirm it. The bone, a human thighbone, he thought, had been discovered in the belly of a railroad tank car that typically transported raw soybean oil to various refinery centers across the country.

The tank car had a thermostat system that maintained a certain temperature in order to prevent the soybean oil from solidifying. It had malfunctioned, and the oil, approximately four feet deep in that particular car, had dried out. Railroad authorities had sidetracked the car. It had sat there for approximately six months and needed to be placed back into operation. However, the dried residue first had to be removed. The only way to do that was for someone to enter the car with a pressure washer and blast it out through the drain holes in the bottom of the car. That they did.

The workers turned the powerful hoses on the sticky, dark brown material and began to break it up. As it broke apart, they flushed it through the drain holes and into barrels to be transported away from the site. Approximately halfway down into the hardened muck, they saw a brown object about twenty inches long that looked like a piece of a tree limb. When they examined it more closely, they called police.

When I saw the thighbone, I understood why they had not recognized it at first as a human bone. It was dark brown in color. The color was a result of sitting in the soybean oil for so long. Bone is porous and will take on the color of the environment around it. Secondly, the femur had an old, dramatic fracture near the mid shaft that had not been treated properly by a medical doctor and had healed out of alignment, giving the bone an irregular shape. Its appearance suggested that the person may not have visited a doctor at all.

The detective asked if I would go down into the tank car and take a closer look at what seemed to the workers to be other bone fragments. Reluctantly, I agreed. The only problem was that there was just one way in and one way out of the tank car: through the hole at the top of the car—the hole that got smaller and smaller as I got closer and closer to it.

I suited up in the oversized yellow slicker the detective provided for me. Then the assistants hooked me up in an apparatus positioned between my legs and up my back and arms, similar perhaps to a parachute harness, which was then attached to the cable on which they would lower me into the tank. They began to lower me inch by inch into the tank car; with every foot I went down, it got darker and darker inside the car and smelled sweeter and sweeter. The dried soybean oil gave off a heady scent reminiscent of old cotton candy.

When I reached the bottom of the car, for only the second time in my life I felt extremely claustrophobic. The other time had been a few years earlier when I had climbed down into a large, fourteen-foot-deep water storage tank, or cistern, located in downtown Baton Rouge between the old military barracks there. It dated to the early nineteenth century and was not known to exist until discovered by accident one day. Naturally, being the curious person I am, I had to document its interior. I decided I was not so curious this time and quickly went to work. I pulled my flashlight from my pocket and directed its powerful beam at various points inside the car. The cleanup work had left pockets of soft soybean residue here and there, interspersed with lumps of hardened material, which made maneuvering with any degree of certainty almost impossible. Added to that was the puppetlike control the cable that lowered me into the car had over my every movement.

Needless to say, my assessment would be brief. As I glanced around inside the car, I saw fragments of human bones everywhere: other long bones, a hipbone, a scapula—all lodged in the soybean matrix. I gently tugged at one of the bones; it would not budge. I knew that recovery of the remains would take place only by softening the material with the water sprayer the workers had already been using.

I motioned for the men above to raise me from the car, and I relished the relief I felt as I breathed fresh air again. We decided that the cleaning crew was better prepared than we were to remove the remaining material. They continued to work with caution and did an excellent job of removing the rest of the bones with little if any damage.

Once we were back at the laboratory with the remains, we determined that approximately two-thirds of a human skeleton was recovered from the car. However, only a few fragments of skull bones and teeth were found. The skeletal remains represented a male approximately thirty-five to forty-five years of age. This assessment was based on the shape of the hipbone and the appearance of its auricular surface.

The anterior-posterior bowing of the femoral shaft suggested he was white, though race could not be determined conclusively without a major portion of the skull, which we did not have.

One of the questions that needed to be answered was how long had the remains been in the tank car: two months? six months? a year? longer? No tissue adhered to the bones. This suggested a minimum time since death of at least six months to a year. Also, some of the remains were missing. If they were not in the tank car or in the barrels of residue from the tank car (which had been searched thoroughly), where were they? At the bottom of the car were the large drainage openings where soybean oil, or any liquid for that matter, could easily be removed from the car on arrival at its destination. Company records on the tank car noted that it had been almost ten years since the car had been refurbished in the early 1990s. That left a window of opportunity of several years when the person could have crawled inside the car or been placed there by someone else. Though no evidence of foul play was found on the recovered bones, crucial bones often associated with foul play, such as those of the skull, were never found.

The broken and healed thighbone led to some speculation that perhaps this person was a hobo, someone who rode the rails on a regular basis. For some unknown reason, he may have become trapped inside the car, unable to get out. We may never find out who he was or what happened to him, but his biological profile has been placed in our IDA database with the hope of sending him home some day.

As for me, I will save any future descents into the belly of the beast for the next generation.

13

Imaging Resources, Cold Cases, and the IDA Database

S OME of the services the FACES Laboratory provides to agencies all across the country include efforts to clear up images captured on video cameras. One such image was brought to our laboratory by the Bureau of Alcohol, Tobacco, and Firearms (ATF). A suspected arsonist was setting fires in abandoned houses. Though no one had been hurt yet, the ATF was very concerned that someone might end up dying if the perpetrator were not identified and stopped. Bureau agents brought a video to our lab, and imaging specialist Eileen Barrow provided assistance in clearing up the frame that included a somewhat blurred image of the alleged perpetrator. A video camera had been placed at a strategic point in the neighborhood where the fires had been occurring and had captured someone setting a fire and then walking away from it. However, his face was not clear enough to publicize because of the distance involved.

Eileen provided the ATF agents with an enhanced image. That image was shown on television stations in the area when an acquaintance of the perpetrator was watching TV in a local establishment. The alleged perpetrator just happened to walk through the door, and the acquaintance recognized him as the person on TV, saying, "Hey, man, that's you." The alleged perpetrator bolted, but with the help of concerned citizens he was caught, at which time he confessed to setting the fires. Eileen's image of him was close enough for the acquaintance to recognize him. We left the rest up to the law. FIGURE 27 shows the video frame, Eileen's enhancement, and the perpetrator's photo.

As illustrated earlier, one service offered by our laboratory is three-dimensional clay facial reconstruction to identify someone when all other ef-

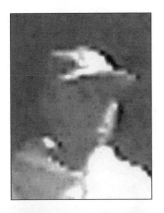

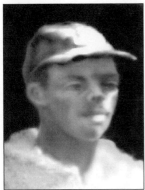

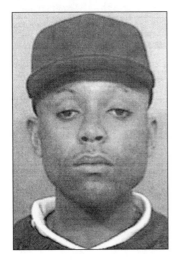

FIGURE 27.
Enhancement of arsonist's video image

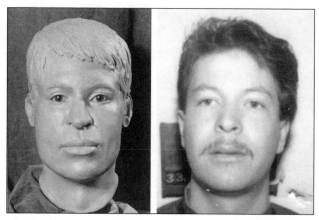

FIGURE 28.
Facial reconstruction and photograph of identified man

forts have failed. One such case from out of state provides an example of
how such images can be successful in identifying someone. FIGURE 28
shows the facial reconstruction that Eileen Barrow prepared for Nevada
authorities in 2001 and the person who was eventually identified. Nevada
law enforcement groups publicized the image throughout their general
area, but they had no positive results. In the summer of 2003, they decided to revisit the cold case and publicized it once again. Immediately,
two women called the authorities and said they thought that the image
looked like their brother who had been missing for several years. When
asked why they had not responded to the publicity of the image in 2001,
they explained that they had been out of the country at the time.

The sisters had held onto an old baseball cap that their brother had
loved. Analysts extracted DNA from the sweat stains on the cap and
matched it to the DNA recovered from his bones. A positive match
proved the man's identity, and his sisters were able to bury their brother
and go on with their lives.

Publicizing the three-dimensional reconstructions for such cases is of utmost importance. We are still hoping that such publicity works in one of
the oldest cases for which we have developed a three-dimensional image.

In 1986, the body of a young white female was found floating in Lake

Pontchartrain in St. Tammany Parish in southeastern Louisiana close to New Orleans. She had a plastic bag over her head and was weighted down with several pounds of material. She was not identified at the time and was buried as a Jane Doe in the paupers' section of a local cemetery.

Detective Marco Dema asked for our help in exhuming her body in 2003. An inquiry had come from out of state on this cold case, and the possibility existed that we might get a positive identification. That possibility led to the judge's order to exhume the victim's body.

We arrived at the cemetery early that summer morning and watched as the backhoe operator removed the soil foot by foot and then inch by inch as he got closer and closer to the body. Records suggested that no casket had been provided and her body had been buried in a body bag. About three and a half feet down into the grave, the backhoe operator hit the remnants of a body bag and then pulled back. Everything else we did that day had to be done by hand. We were thankful for the silty-sandy soil in that area, which made the final recovery work fairly easy.

The body bag had deteriorated somewhat in the sixteen years since the victim had been buried, but small amounts of adipocere and tissue were still present across her skeleton. Her body had fared better than others we had seen that had not been buried that long, thanks in part to the plastic body bag and the type of soil in which she was buried.

After hours of painstaking work, we recovered her body and transported it to the FACES Lab for analysis. The results of the original autopsy had provided incredible details about this young woman, details that should have led to a positive identification more than sixteen years earlier. She was a small, white female, approximately eighteen to twenty-five years of age. She had been strangled before being placed in the lake. Also, she had breast implants that were revealed at autopsy. Finally, she was more than three months pregnant when she was murdered.

If dental charts were made at the time of her autopsy, they no longer existed, nor could any dental x-rays be found. We could certainly create a dental chart to compare to the missing woman from out of state and could also take x-rays of her teeth to be held in perpetuity in case she was not the young woman in question.

By comparing the new chart we made for the young woman with the dental records of the woman from out of state, we determined that she was not the same woman. That young woman had fillings in certain teeth where ours did not. In fact, the woman found in Lake Pontchartrain had no fillings in her perfect teeth. You cannot take away a filling without replacing it with another restoration of some kind. You could replace it with a crown, a false tooth, or a new filling, but a filled tooth cannot revert to being a perfect tooth. Enamel cannot rejuvenate itself. The woman from the lake also had no wisdom teeth, the last molar in each of the four tooth quadrants. She was either born without them (what we call congenital absence) or may have had them removed. Though we definitively eliminated our victim as a match for the young woman missing from out of state by comparing dental charts and x-rays, hundreds and hundreds of other young women are missing. One of them might be our victim.

A very important finding in our case that had not been noted at autopsy was the fact that our victim had experienced major trauma to her hips. She had been in some kind of an accident in the past, such as an automobile accident, or she may have been kicked very hard in the pelvis. Those bones were in the process of healing when she was killed. The trauma was severe enough that she clearly would have to have been hospitalized for a time.

Our next task was to provide Eileen Barrow with all of the background she needed to create a clay image for the young woman. FIGURE 29 is a photo of the facial reconstruction that Eileen completed. Though advertised in the New Orleans area in 2003, it still has not resulted in a positive identification. It has now been nineteen years since this young woman's body was found, but with the help of the public we may send her home.

Cases such as this one will become more and more prominent as we reevaluate them and enter them into our new IDA database. The database represents an ambitious effort on the part of the LSU FACES Laboratory to provide comprehensive, cutting-edge information on two groups of victims in our state: the more than sixty cases in our lab for

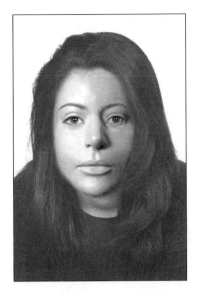

FIGURE 29.
Facial reconstruction of strangling victim

which we have been unable to establish the victim's identity (out of the hundreds on which we have worked in the last twenty-four years) and the many people across our state who are missing.

IDA will contain biological and DNA profiles on all of Louisiana's missing and unidentified cases for which we are able to obtain data. In a cooperative effort with the Louisiana State Police Crime Laboratory and the North Louisiana Crime Laboratory (NLCL) in Shreveport, we are compiling computer files like no others in the country. DNA samples from unidentified cases and from family members of missing people will be recorded by FACES and the NLCL. The DNA data will also become part of a larger database being established by the FBI to assist in cold case analysis.

Research associate Beth Bassett and I are currently traveling across Louisiana to gather personal profile information and DNA samples for these cases. Ideally, we plan to add every new case that comes up. By doing so, we hope to make positive identifications of the unidentified and missing more likely. As the first comprehensive database of its kind in the country, IDA could become a model for other interested agencies.

Finally, though our work with IDA has only just started, we have already positively identified the remains of a young man who had been on our unidentified list for three years.

Under Siege

SOMEONE was killing Louisiana's women. In fact, women were being murdered at an alarming rate, and many of them were dying in the shadow of Louisiana's capitol of Baton Rouge. In 2002, local and national media attention became focused on a situation that some law enforcement agents and I had been concerned about for more than a decade. Women from all walks of life were being murdered in a rather compressed area of our state: college students, recent college graduates, young and mature professional women, and prostitutes.

By 2002, the murders were coming closer and closer together and had totaled more than twenty-five by some estimates. By that time, law enforcement agencies also had the technology that would tie some of them together: DNA sampling. When three murders that had occurred within a period of a few months of one another were linked by DNA in 2002, "serial killer" became a buzz word in the news. The magic number three was the minimum number needed for authorities to assign the term "serial killer" to a series of deaths.

As law enforcement agents, investigative reporters, and others began to dig deeper into the past, they discovered case after case that might be linked to what was thought to be a lone murderer. Eventually, authorities determined that the killer was operating not just in Baton Rouge but in an area that encompassed hundreds of square miles and affected families in more than seven parishes.

"Serial killer" is a descriptor reserved for one of the most heinous of criminals and has been associated with such names as Ted Bundy, John Wayne Gacy, Jeffrey Dahmer, and Henry Lee Lucas. The forecast was ominous.

The fear in the eyes of women across the city of Baton Rouge and surrounding communities became palpable. Law enforcement groups
formed a task force that included sheriffs' departments, police departments, the Office of the Attorney General, the Louisiana State Police, the
U.S. attorney, and the FBI. As time passed, the killer struck again, as
though nothing and no one could stop his wanton desire to destroy
women and their families.

The perpetrator was profiled as being probably a white male under
the age of forty. Further corroboration of that description appeared in the
news when a truck driver saw who he thought was a white male with a
woman in a truck that had exited the interstate at the very exit where one
of the victims was later found.

The streets became deserted. Even in the daytime, the usual hundreds
of female joggers and walkers disappeared from along the streets of Baton
Rouge and from around the lakes at Louisiana State University. Women
bought dogs and guns, many guns. Women who had never planned to
own a gun in their lives started taking target practice classes. Pepper spray
was on the key chain of almost every woman in the city. Most of them
held it close to their chests when they exited their vehicles or walked to
their doors. They did not fully realize that it offered little, if any, true pro-
tection and might actually hurt their chance of survival if they got it in
their own eyes accidentally while trying to spray a would-be assailant. My
husband bought two canisters of the spray, one for his mom and one for
me. Knowing that I had been raised in a family of Tasmanian devils, he
tried to make light of the situation by suggesting that I offer mine to any
potential assailant with the idea of leveling the playing field. But I knew
that he was concerned.

Self-defense classes sprang up all over Baton Rouge, and for the first
time in my life, I felt unsafe in my adopted city. I had been raised in a
gun-totin' family and was comfortable with one, knowing I could shoot
anyone if someone were threatening my life and I actually had access to a
gun. Though I refused to be paralyzed by fear, as some of my friends
were, I had to admit that going out for my morning walk seemed more of
a challenge than usual. Routinely, I had varied my walking route and had

never used a walkman or anything that would distract me, but the slightest sound behind me now made me a little crazy. I consoled myself with the idea that the killer mainly targeted younger women quite a distance from my neighborhood. However, no one knew exactly how many of the women who had been murdered in the Baton Rouge area over the last twenty years or so had actually been killed by this monster, and very few had seen what I had seen: the results of his rage.

Every white male in the area became suspect. DNA swabs were taken from more than a thousand men. Rumors spread like wildfire, and upstanding reputations became threatened at the slightest hint of involvement. Thousands of phone tips went to the task force. Weirdos came out in full force, and false claims of personal attacks took an untold number of hours to address. Finally, after what seemed an eternity, a series of events began to fall into place in 2003 and then again in 2004 that would result in the arrest and subsequent indictments of not one but two serial killer suspects, both male, operating totally independent of one another—one black and one white.

My role as a forensic anthropologist would be ancillary in some cases and in others more direct. Jim Churchman, director of physical evidence at the Louisiana State Police Crime Laboratory, made sure that I was invited to the initial meeting of law enforcement agents and other groups assembled in Baton Rouge to address the crisis. The participants from all across south Louisiana began to discuss different cases as a prelude to the establishment of a formal task force, and I realized that I had consulted on many of the cases mentioned.

My personal experience with murders of local women went back more than twenty years, and the identity of the perpetrator was still unknown in many cases. In fact, some of the victims were still missing. For years, various officers and I had discussed the similarities in some of the cases and how it seemed that at least two different persons were responsible for these dastardly deeds. After several young professional women became victims of the killer or killers and their bodies were discovered soon enough after death to provide DNA evidence, investigators became encouraged that the cases might be solved. This breakthrough was more significant than many realized, as news accounts of serial killer cases across the country had shown that such cases could take more than a decade to solve or might never be solved at all.

My account of certain events related to the cases on which I worked will provide the public with an understanding of my role as a forensic anthropologist in that series of events that crippled our city and surrounding cities for years. Not all of the cases reported by the media came through my laboratory, but quite a few of the murders of women in south Louisiana in the last twenty years, especially in the parishes surrounding East Baton Rouge, were cases that ended up in my laboratory for one reason or another.

As noted earlier, forensic anthropologists may be "invited" to consult on a case in Louisiana, whether the death is from homicide, suicide, natural causes, or unknown causes. Oftentimes, our role is to assist with a positive identification. Other times, we are asked to evaluate trauma.

In any death case, if a possible, or putative, identification is available, that identification still has to be confirmed through some means. In the past, and still in many cases today, antemortem dental records represent one of the quickest ways to confirm identification. We always take full body x-rays of any case that passes through our laboratory, regardless of whether it is a recent death or there are only skeletal remains. Afterwards, we take dental x-rays of the person in case antemortem x-rays become available for comparison.

If the person has been dead for only a short period of time, anywhere from a few hours to a few weeks, we may play a role in the initial stages of the case. We may help with body recovery. On some occasions, the body will be brought to the FACES Lab at LSU, where we will assist investigators by completing the initial x-rays. Additionally, we might attend the autopsy. There, as a general rule, we simply observe while the forensic pathologist, the medical doctor who typically determines cause and manner of death, conducts a full-scale autopsy.

Our role in the case may end there, or it may continue, depending on preliminary findings by the pathologist. Through consultation with the law enforcement agency involved, we may request that the pathologist extract different parts of the body to aid in identification and/or to examine those elements more closely for trauma. This is especially true if the body is in an advanced stage of decomposition where putrefactive tissue needs to be removed to have a better understanding of the exact nature of the trauma. Such extractions may make the layman uncomfortable, but as an advocate for the victim, my role in the case is to provide as much information as possible about what happened to that person. For justice to prevail, I have to make tough decisions about such matters. Legal statutes allow for examination and retention of any body part deemed evidence by the coroner and germane to the resolution of a case.

In some cases over the years, I have been asked to assist in identification when the person has been dead for less than forty-eight hours. The public might assume that so soon after death the individual could easily be identified visually by a family member or friend—if only that were always the case.

So many things play a role in the initial identification process: environment, time of year, climate, trauma, and covering over the body all contribute to the condition of a set of remains. In certain instances in our subtropical climate, individuals are totally unrecognizable after only twenty-four hours. Their decomposition can be so advanced that even trying to x-ray their teeth offers unique challenges. If trauma of any kind has been inflicted against the person, the difficulty level of the case analysis rises dramatically.

If a week or more passes before a body is discovered, certain other challenges face the investigators and the forensic pathologist, making the role of a forensic anthropologist more important in the investigation. By the time two weeks have passed, especially if the body has lain out on the surface during summer and fall, that body can be almost totally skeletonized, resulting in a situation where the forensic pathologist can offer little if any assistance.

As persons trained in analysis of the human skeleton, forensic anthropologists can provide the preliminary profile of age, sex, race, height, trauma analysis, and an estimation of time since death for those cases on which we are consulted. Even if other evidence at the scene suggests the identity of the person, positive identification still must be confirmed.

My history with missing and murdered women in the Baton Rouge area began with the case of Eleanor Parker, a beautiful young college student who disappeared in 1982 while I was still a graduate student in anthropology. Eleanor's car was found abandoned a few days after she disappeared, but she was never found. Even after almost a quarter of a century, her name immediately comes to my mind when human remains of an unidentified white female are discovered. In such cases, we compare the unidentified female with Eleanor's biological and dental profiles.

In 1985, a few years after Eleanor's disappearance, LSU Ph.D. student Melissa Montz was reported missing after she had gone out jogging early one morning before class. I knew Melissa well enough to say "Hello" when we saw each other in the hallways, because our departments were in the same building. I also knew that Melissa was very athletic and usually jogged several miles a day. Additionally, I felt in my heart that we would get her body. Hundreds of volunteers combed the nearby ditches, the LSU lakes, and other areas stretching for miles around the campus, retracing her known jogging routes. Flyers were posted everywhere. Nothing like that had happened so close to the campus before.

One Saturday morning, almost seven weeks after Melissa disappeared, I was at a craft festival when my name was called out over the public address system. My husband was the only person in the world who knew that I was there. Of course, it made me nervous. The call, however, was from Dr. Douglas Owsley, my boss at the time. "Mary, they've found her," he said. "Can you come to the lab?" He didn't have to say who "her" was. We had just had a conversation about Melissa the evening before in the lab.

A golfer on the LSU golf course saw a dog with what appeared to be a human leg bone. He called the police. Most of the rest of Melissa's body was discovered adjacent to Nicholson Drive near the LSU campus and contiguous with the golf course. Because she had been missing for several weeks, crucial evidence had been lost. The decomposition process had done its job. Only skeletal remains were available for our assessment. Yet they told us who she was and what had happened to her. Her killer has never been found.

The years between 1986 and 1992 were fairly quiet in terms of the murders of local women. However, 1992 would be different. Hurricane Andrew arrived in the summer with a vengeance and helped to accelerate the decomposition of the body of Connie Warner. Connie was a forty-one-year-old white female who had disappeared from her home late one evening in Zachary, Louisiana, a small city just north of Baton Rouge in East Baton Rouge Parish. She had been missing for three weeks when her remains were discovered in a ditch in an industrial area of Baton Rouge. I was called to the scene, where I met Dr. Lamar Meek, a forensic entomologist. He had been asked to estimate how long the body had been in the ditch. I was asked to profile the skeleton. Our evaluation linked the remains to Connie. We identified her through dental records and described what had happened to her. Her murderer was never discovered.

In 1997, Eugenie Boisfontaine disappeared. Eugenie was an avid walker and was often seen at different times of day walking around the LSU lakes and up and down Stanford Avenue, where she lived. I had seen her myself on my way to school, a rather serious-looking young woman who seemed very concentrated on her walks. She was in the midst of planning a trip to Europe when she disappeared. A few days after she disappeared, her keys and driver's license were found by a jogger near the edge of one of the LSU lakes. Her body was found weeks later near a bayou in Iberville Parish (which is immediately adjacent to East Baton Rouge Parish). Eugenie's body was first autopsied and then brought to my lab by Iberville Parish authorities. The advanced stage of decomposition had obscured crucial evidence during the initial evaluation of her remains, evidence we were able to document once we prepared her for analysis. Authorities were very glad they brought her to our lab. Once again, we helped to identify Eugenie, and we described what had happened to her. Her killer was not found.

In 1999, Hardee Moseley Schmidt disappeared early one morning when she was out for her usual morning jog. Her body was discovered two days later in St. James Parish, a few miles south of Baton Rouge, in a watery grave. Detectives asked for my assistance in identifying her, and I met them at Earl K. Long Hospital in Baton Rouge. Her body was being held there temporarily before transfer to a laboratory where she was to be autopsied the next day. Hardee's identification and case analysis would prove to be a challenge for a number of reasons, not the least of which was the fact that her body had been dumped in a watery environment. We attended her autopsy, helped to identify her, and assisted with evaluating what had happened to her.

In Hardee's case, we worked tirelessly around the clock to provide crucial positive identification confirmation and to assess other evidence regarding her remains. I then rushed to the funeral home just minutes prior to her wake to make sure that everything associated with her body could be placed in her casket. Many never knew the extent to which we went to ensure the family had all of her body for burial. Hardee's killer remained unknown.

In January of 2000, we received two cases of women whose bodies had been dumped: Lillian Robinson, a black female, fifty-two, who was found in St. Martin Parish in a watery grave, and Robin Gremillion, a white female, twenty-eight, whose body was discovered floating in one of the LSU lakes. In both cases, we attended the autopsies, helped to identify the women, and checked their bodies for evidence of trauma. The perpetrator or perpetrators were unknown.

In February 2000, I received a phone call from Yancy Guerin. Yancy, a coroner's investigator for Iberville Parish, had some bones he wanted me to examine. They had been found on the river side of the levee in his parish, and he wanted to determine whether they were human. He presented me with an entire lower leg, a human leg. He thought they were human but others disagreed. "Yancy," I said, "we need to find the rest of this body."

"I agree, Mary. Can you help?" It just so happened that the spring semester at LSU had only recently begun, and I had a group of fifteen graduate students eager to do a field recovery. Off we went to the levee, where I met an investigator from the Louisiana State Police Crime Lab. Adam Becnel walked down the concrete-covered levee that cold, sunny day with a friendly smile. His scrubbed-clean appearance and youthful look were deceiving. I had encountered a tenacious, hardworking investigator who would take in everything I said and prove to be a staunch ally for years to come. Best of all, he readily accepted that once the scene was turned over to me, how to proceed would indeed be my call. Adam and I instantly became friends and have subsequently conducted research projects together.

Before we began the search and recovery of the victim behind the levee, Adam and my assistants took copious photographs of several items that were obviously noteworthy from the moment we arrived on the scene. After that, we began to fan out and systematically look for other remains. We flagged everything we found and photographed them in place, or in situ. Once we were satisfied that we had found all of the remains we were going to find that day, we mapped the bones and finally picked them up. The bones were widespread and our final map would show that their distribution ran parallel to the levee on the river side and stretched for a distance twice the length of a football field.

Though the body was completely skeletonized, I could tell Yancy that we had the remains of a young black female over twenty-five and that she had lain out in the elements for several months. I could also provide him with details of what had happened to her. Through good ole detective work, Yancy eventually found hospital records that helped us identify the victim. She was Joyce Williams, a young black woman who had been missing for several months, since the fall of 1999. Her killer remained at large.

In November 2000, FACES Lab personnel assisted with the recovery of Marilyn Nevils's body from behind the levee on River Road in East Baton Rouge Parish. A young man walking his dog had found her there. Marilyn was a white female, age thirty-eight. She had been dead for only six days or so when she was discovered. We helped to identify her and reported on what had happened to her. Her killer was unknown.

The killings came more and more frequently over the next few years. Some of them came through my lab for a variety of reasons. The skeletal remains of Christine Moore, a young black LSU graduate student, were found in May 2002, on River Road in East Baton Rouge Parish near a small pond and church only a few miles from LSU. Though her body was skeletonized, we were able to recover her remains, assist with her identification, and evaluate her skeleton for evidence of what happened to her. Her killer was unknown.

A short time later in 2002, Pam Kinamore, a white forty-four-year-old antique store owner, disappeared from her home in Baton Rouge late one night. Her body was found in Whiskey Bay, an area off Interstate 10 between Baton Rouge and Lafayette. It was near the same area where Carrie Yoder's body would be found in 2003. Carrie was a twenty-seven-year-old Ph.D. student at LSU who lived just outside the south gates of the main campus. It was believed, that she, too, had been abducted from her home. Both bodies came through the FACES Lab.

By 2004, still others had been handled through our lab: Donna Bennett Johnston and Johnnie Mae Williams among them. Donna was a white female a little over forty years old, and Johnnie Mae was a black female a little over thirty years old.

Some of the murdered women did not become part of our casework at the FACES Lab. In 2002, Charlotte Murray Pace was murdered in her home not far from the LSU campus. We did not work on Murray's case. Also, Gina Wilson Green, who had been killed in her home in fall 2001, was not a case that came through my lab. Coincidentally, Pace, Green, and Boisfontaine all lived within one or two blocks of one another on Stanford Avenue near LSU at one time. Murray had just moved from there when she was murdered at her home in Sharlo, a subdivision in south Baton Rouge.

Other prominent cases highlighted in the media that were not part of our caseload include those of Geralyn DeSoto (who was murdered in her home in West Baton Rouge Parish), Katherine Hall (found in East Baton Rouge Parish), and Trineisha Dené Colomb (found in Lafayette Parish approximately sixty miles from Baton Rouge). As many as ten or more other women who died between 1994 and 2004 were cases that had not come through my lab.

During those years, missing women also became part of our caseload. In Zachary, Louisiana, a nurse, Randi Mebruer, who had been missing from her home since 1998, became a person we all felt we knew. Randi was a beautiful young nurse with a little boy. When a neighbor saw the little boy out riding his tricycle alone early one morning, police were called to what has been described in the news as a gruesome scene. Over the years, we have assisted in digging up front yards covered with cement and draining an entire lake searching for her body. She has not yet been found. She lived just a block or so from Connie Warner, who had been killed in 1992 and dumped in Baton Rouge.

Mary Ann Fowler is another woman missing from Baton Rouge. On December 24, 2002, Mary Ann was abducted from in front of a sandwich shop on Highway 417 where she had stopped for a quick bite to eat. On multiple occasions we have examined isolated bones found in the general vicinity where she was abducted. Like Mebreur, Fowler has not been found.

I was witnessing an unbelievably long list of victims whose families cried out for justice. Finally, in what seemed like a miracle, evidence gathered from some of the cases pointed toward a particular suspect. That suspect was Derrick Todd Lee, a thirty-four-year-old black male. Lee was arrested in May 2003 and tried in 2004 in West Baton Rouge Parish for the murder of Geralyn DeSoto, the recent LSU graduate who had plans to enter graduate school shortly. In that case, Lee was found guilty of second-degree murder and was sentenced to life in prison without parole. News accounts documented how DNA linked Lee to that case, the same evidence that, according to other news accounts, linked him to the deaths of Murray Pace, Pam Kinamore, Gina Green, Carrie Yoder, Dené Colomb, and Randi Mebreur.

In the fall of 2004, Derrick Todd Lee was tried and convicted in East Baton Rouge Parish for the murder of Murray Pace. Hist first-degree murder conviction resulted in his being sentenced to death for her murder.

Lee's conviction came on the heels of another arrest in the summer of 2004, when authorities had gotten another lucky break. After Lee had been arrested in 2003, the murders of women in the Baton Rouge area had continued, including those of Donna Bennett Johnston and Johnnie Mae Williams. With Lee in jail, it was as though the other killer that detectives and I thought all along must be out there was saying, "Hey, what about me? I'm still here. Look what I can do."

According to news accounts, a tire track left at the scene where the body of Donna Bennett Johnston was found led law enforcement agents to Sean Gillis, a soft-spoken forty-one-year-old white male. Out of the blue, Gillis confessed to multiple murders, including those of Hardee Moseley Schmidt, Ann Bryan, Joyce Williams, Donna Bennett Johnston, Katherine Hall, Marilyn Nevils, Lillian Robinson, and Johnnie Mae Williams. Gillis was arraigned and indicted for the murder of Donna Bennett Johnston. At his arraignment, he pleaded not guilty. As of this writing, he awaits trial for her murder.

Within a brief period, two serial killer suspects had been identified and arrested, their alleged victims of various ages, races, and socioeconomic circumstances. Those victims all left behind grieving family members and friends who will not rest until justice is served for every victim. Various trials for the two suspects will take years.

For the families of the murder victims, the pain and anger will never go away completely. For those law enforcement personnel and others who worked so diligently to solve these cases, public criticism of their efforts sometimes was hard to handle, though the officers often understood. Those of us at the FACES Lab who have been involved in some of the cases have been forever changed by the experience.

Finally, for the families of Eleanor Parker, Randi Mebruer, Mary Ann Fowler, and other women who remain missing, but who may not have been mentioned in this account, we at the LSU FACES Lab are forever vigilant in our efforts to help find them. We constantly watch for any leads that could someday help bring their loved ones home.

15

Space Shuttle Columbia

O N Saturday, February 1, 2003, at about 8:00 A.M., I remembered that I planned to go outside my house in Baton Rouge to see if I could view the space shuttle *Columbia* going by overhead. It was returning to earth that morning after a sixteen-day mission with its seven astronauts. I never saw it. Soon thereafter, I heard the unbelievable news that it had broken apart in flames. News accounts reported that NASA had lost communication with *Columbia* somewhere over California at an altitude above 200,000 feet. *Columbia* was thought to be traveling at six times the speed of sound.

Ultimately, we would learn that debris from the ship fell to the ground over hundreds of miles of countryside, mainly in Texas and Louisiana. Witnesses had heard a big bang and saw flames in the sky.

All seven aboard were lost. Among them were six American astronauts: Michael Anderson, David Brown, Kalpana Chawla, Laurel Clark, Rick Husband, and William McCool. The seventh was Ilan Ramon, Israel's first astronaut.

Our country was in shock once again. We were still reeling from the September 11 attacks just a year and a half before and simply could not believe a tragedy of such magnitude could occur to our astronauts, whose smiling, happy faces we had all seen over and over again as they headed for the shuttle and for the stars.

Prior to the shuttle disaster, I had only recently completed the procedures for joining a federal disaster team known as the Disaster Mortuary Operational Response Team (DMORT). At the time, DMORT was a part of the Department of Health and Human Services. We are now with Homeland Security under the Federal Emergency Management Agency (FEMA).

DMORT membership is restricted to certain professionals across the country who possess the skills required to aid the federal government in mass disasters. The teams are made up of pathologists, nurses, hazardous materials experts, funeral home directors, forensic odontologists, forensic anthropologists, and other specialists who can assist with the recovery and identification of victims of mass disasters including natural disasters, such as hurricanes, tornadoes, and floods, and man-made disasters such as the September 11 terrorist attacks.

Though I was not a member of DMORT in 2001 and, because of that, could not assist at the World Trade Center, the Pennsylvania hillside crash site, or the Pentagon, I decided that I wanted to join DMORT in the off chance that I could assist if and when a time I might be needed came again.

DMORT teams are assigned to regions. Region 6 includes Louisiana, Texas, Oklahoma, New Mexico, and Arkansas. If a disaster occurs within our region or any other region where our expertise is needed, we must be ready to deploy on a moment's notice, similar to the National Guard. Our bags must always be packed and ready to go with enough clothing and other items to last for a minimum of two weeks.

Little did I know that I would be needed so soon. Several days had passed since the shuttle accident had occurred, and no word had come out of Texas about what was happening there. Like any citizen, I looked for news about the crash and wondered what condition the bodies might be in if they were found. Everywhere I went, people asked me if I knew what was happening in Texas. I gave them an honest answer: "I have no idea."

Out of the blue, late on the afternoon of February 7, six days after the accident, Chuck Smith reached me in the FACES Lab. I had known Chuck for twenty years or more when he worked as a senior coroner's investigator at the local coroner's office. Currently, he is a deputy commander for Region 6 of the DMORT teams. "Mary, we need you and we need you now," he said. "Can you come today?"

I said, "Sure I can. What about Ginny Listi?" Ginny had joined the DMORT team at the same time I had.

"Let me check and get back with you," Chuck said. "We already have

Julie Powers coming out of New Mexico." I knew Julie. She and I had often chatted at the annual conference of the American Academy of Forensic Sciences, to which we both belonged. Julie also had worked at the World Trade Center disaster. Chuck called back within a few minutes and said, "Yes, we need you both."

Ginny and I hurried home and packed and hit the road, making arrangements for classes to be handled the next week by teaching assistants and others. It was early evening before we left Baton Rouge, and we knew we had at least a five-and-a-half- or six-hour trip ahead of us to reach Lufkin, a city in east Texas. Most DMORT personnel were stationed in Lufkin, though it was not the major command center for the entire recovery effort.

In Chuck's brief conversation with me, he had mentioned a little town of approximately eleven hundred people right out of my past, Hemphill, Texas. Hemphill was the destination of probably thousands of people involved in the recovery effort. It was the command center where everyone came together, representing more than eighty agencies. Hemphill was also the birthplace of my father and his father and his father before him. Though my father left Hemphill when he was fairly young, I would later learn that Hemphill's first jail was built by bricks from the kiln of my great-grandfather, Kip Huffman. I would also learn that the town library now carried the Huffman name. What a strange feeling came over me. I had only been to Hemphill once in my life, when I was about eight years old. I never thought I would ever go there again.

Chuck had only briefly described why our expertise was needed. The shuttle debris was thought to be strewn over possibly hundreds of miles of heavily wooded area, a major portion of it in a region known as the Big Thicket Forest. Thousands of volunteers and professionals had been working nonstop to help find the astronauts and shuttle debris. Small problem: in any wooded area where you have animals, you will have animal bones. Bones were being found everywhere, and DMORT needed forensic anthropologists to determine if those remains were human or nonhuman.

Reaching our destination that first night after midnight and securing a fitful night's sleep on the last bed in the motel, I awoke the next morning with apprehension. It was very cold in February in east Texas, and it was raining. Our management support team was domiciled at the hotel where we were staying. That team took care of all of our needs and assigned us to various geographical areas. Ginny went with a team to a staging site approximately an hour or so away from Hemphill, and Julie and I were assigned to Hemphill.

Hemphill was an hour's drive from Lufkin, but there were no hotel rooms in Hemphill. Though situated near the edge of Toledo Bend, one of the most beautiful fishing spots in all of America, few hotels had ever sprung up in the area. Those that were there filled to capacity immediately after the disaster occurred.

I met some wonderful professionals in my first deployment under DMORT. I had worked with Chuck Smith for years in Baton Rouge but did not realize until this deployment that he had essential computer skills with Global Positioning System (GPS) software. Those skills would prove invaluable to all of the teams working in the Big Thicket and other areas where evidence was discovered. He provided data that were vital to the success of the operation and that saved many of us from getting totally lost in deep, thick woods as we rendezvoused with various teams to identify the material in question.

With Julie Powers and me as the two forensic anthropologists in our area, our team in Hemphill also consisted of Dr. David Senn, a forensic odontologist from the University of Texas Health Science Center in San Antonio, and Dr. Corinne Stern, chief medical examiner from El Paso, Texas. We became fast friends as we shared our sorrowful tasks and dubbed ourselves the "Demortologists."

A call to any area to check out remains that had been found by advance teams could mean traveling by vehicle for thirty minutes or more, often in rough-riding Humvees driven by national guardsmen, and then walking through the Big Thicket for miles on end. Each team included agents from the FBI.

Volunteers fell by the wayside. Some twisted their ankles, others twisted their shoulders while fording streams, still others became completely exhausted while trying to overcome the inevitable digestive problems associated with such group gatherings. And still we marched. Luckily, I was used to the woods. I had grown up in a similar area and never lost my love for the outdoors. Though searching for human remains might not seem appealing, I've always considered being outdoors and in the woods one of the benefits of my job.

Little things became so important. The citizens of Hemphill and surrounding communities were phenomenal. They helped to make everyone's stay as pleasant as possible. They even manned a supply center filled with items donated by various companies. They would see me coming and get out the Band-Aids for my blistered heels. My favorite thing they had in stock was free socks—glorious, free, dry socks. I felt so spoiled and fortunate.

The cold got colder, and the rain got wetter. Water filled my boots; branches tore at my face; thick plastic slickers were shredded by the briar thickets we encountered regularly and that could have challenged even the best Brer Rabbit. But our luck held. We were finding what we had come to find.

Each time we returned to the command post after an especially grueling trip into the thicket, my heart would break. There, waiting to thank us, to shake our hands, to tell us how grateful they were for our assistance, were other astronauts, all hoping for news about their comrades and friends. They were thanking me—thanking *me*—when all I wanted to do was thank them for being so brave as to do the things they do. They had ultimate sadness in their eyes and continuing disbelief in their countenance. At some point, being the goober I am, I asked for autographs to keep as mementos of meeting them, which they willingly gave, as well as pictures and patches and shuttle pins.

In the end, we gave them back their friends and comrades, all seven of them. The remains of the astronauts were shipped to Dover, Delaware, for processing and positive identification.

Finally, Ginny and I packed up our gear, said good-bye to all of our new friends, and drove away: away from Hemphill, away from the place

of my father's birth, away from the national news media who were winding down when we parted, and away from the sorrow that clung to everything there like a heavy black mantle. We returned to our regular jobs of
teaching and research and identifying the dead.

Though almost twenty-five years of dealing with death might have made
me immune to such things as the shuttle crash, I am thankful that has
never happened. Each case I receive affects me in some way. Some affect
me more than others.

To this day, when I think about that week in east Texas, it seems almost surreal. Did all of that really happen? Did we really lose our space
pioneers in such a horrible way? Did I actually go into the Big Thicket
and find my way home? Sometimes, late at night, when I cannot sleep
and I sit outside alone, I look toward the heavens, thankful for what I
have and who I am, and I pause to remember our brave and tragic astronauts out among the stars.